Student Record Book

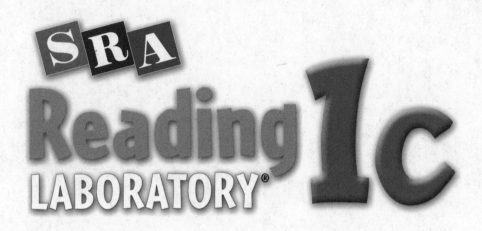

Columbus, Ohio

The McGraw·Hill Companies

SRAonline.com

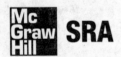 **SRA**

Contents

Letter to Parents

Over the years, millions of children from cities such as New York, London, Chicago, Toronto, Los Angeles, and Sydney have had one thing in common— they have used "the SRA." "The SRA" is what students have often called *SRA Reading Laboratory.* This school year your child will be using SRA's most recent *Reading Laboratory.* This multileveled system of individualized instruction will provide your child with practice in reading comprehension, vocabulary skills, and study skills. In most classrooms, this program will supplement your child's reader, giving him or her extra reinforcement in a wide range of reading-related skills.

SRA Reading Laboratory offers 144 reading selections. These selections include high-interest nonfiction and fiction that cover a wide range of topics. The settings of many of the stories or articles take place in a variety of places around the world. These selections offer enjoyment in reading for the students, as well as providing them with important information that will broaden their understanding of many global concerns, events, and issues. The reading selections are divided into levels. Each level is represented by a different color, and each color is more difficult to read than the previous color. Therefore, when you hear, "Today I started in Blue!" you are learning of a significant accomplishment.

Each selection is accompanied by exercises that test for students' understanding of the selection. Additional exercises provide practice in vocabulary, word building, and study skills. At the beginning of the school year, each student is placed in a level at which he or she can read successfully. The system then allows your child to move through the levels as fast and as far as his or her ability permits.

Students have been using and enjoying *SRA Reading Laboratory* since 1957. You may have used one of the earlier editions yourself! May your knowledge of this most recent edition increase your understanding of your child's reading enjoyment and progress.

The Crow and the Crocodile

by Virginia Brosseit

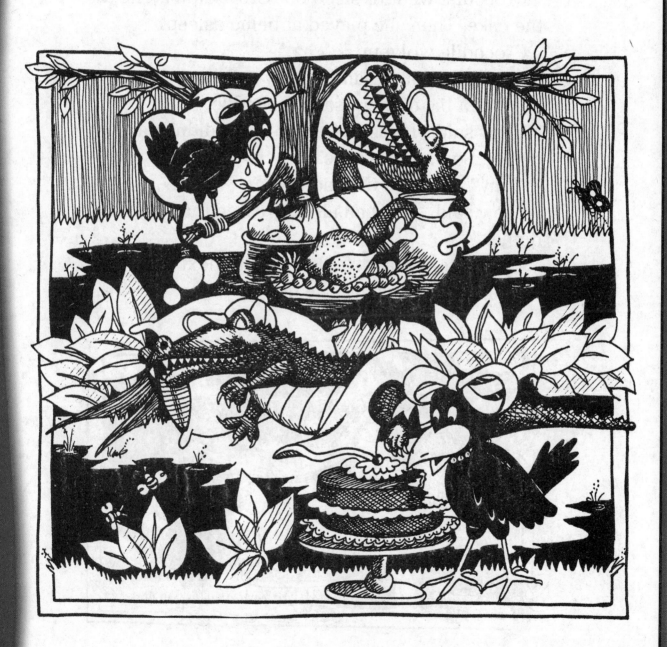

Crow and Crocodile found a big cake.

"Let's share it," said Crow.

Crocodile said, "I want it all."

"Let's sleep," said Crow. "The one who has the best dream gets the cake."

Crocodile went to sleep but Crow didn't. She ate the cake. Then she played at being asleep.

Crocodile woke up.

"What did you dream?" Crow asked.

"I had a big dinner," said Crocodile.

Crow said, "I was there, too, but I didn't eat the dinner. So I ate the cake."

"Why?" shouted Crocodile.

Crow said, "You had already eaten that big dinner."

Crocodile laughed. "All right. But next time I get the cake and you have the dream."

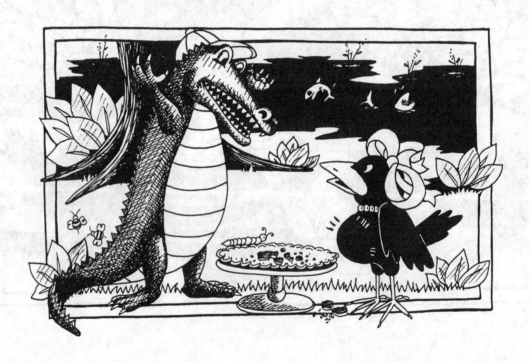

A Read each question. Write *a* or *b*.

1 What is funny about this story?
   a The way Crow gets all the cake
   b The way Crocodile gets his dinner

2 Why did Crocodile go to sleep?
   a Because he wanted the cake
   b Because he was very tired

3 Why did Crow *not* go to sleep?
   a So Crocodile would have to share
   b So she could eat all the cake

4 What did Crocodile eat?
   a Crocodile ate a big dinner.
   b Crocodile didn't eat anything.

5 Why did Crocodile laugh?
   a Because Crow's trick was funny
   b Because Crow's dream was silly

LEARN ABOUT WORDS

B sl + **ow** = **slow**

Look at each row of letters. Add one letter or group of letters from each row to *ow* to make a word. Write the word.

1	gr, dr, sr
2	wh, tr, kn
3	cl, sn, sm + **ow**
4	d, r, j
5	qu, cr, gh

LEARN ABOUT WORDS (continued)

C Read the words you wrote. Which one best fits in each sentence? Write the word.

6 Crocodile didn't _____ where the cake came from.

7 "Did it _____ out of the ground?" he asked.

8 "Maybe it fell out of the sky," said the _____.

9 The white frosting on the cake looked like _____.

10 The cake had a _____ of pink roses on it.

THINK ABOUT IT

D Read the sentences. Which answer tells what *it* means? Write *a* or *b*.

1 Crow found a cake under a tree. She wanted to share *it* with Crocodile. *It* means

   a a tree. **b** a cake.

2 Crocodile thought the frosting looked like snow. He liked *it*. *It* means

   a the frosting. **b** snow.

3 Crocodile had a dream when he took a nap. He told Crow about *it*. *It* means

   a a nap. **b** a dream.

4 "I had a dream about a big dinner. I ate *it* all," Crocodile said. *It* means

   a a big dinner. **b** a dream.

5 Crow played a trick when she ate the cake. Crocodile thought *it* was funny. *It* means

   a a trick. **b** the cake.

Starter Story Record Page

Name _____ Date _____

Power Builder Color _____ Power Builder Number _____

A Comprehension

1 _____ 2 _____ 3 _____ 4 _____ 5 _____

Number Correct [ ]

B, C Learn about Words

1 _____ 6 _____

2 _____ 7 _____

3 _____ 8 _____

4 _____ 9 _____

5 _____ 10 _____

Number Correct [ ]

Think about It

D 1 _____ E 6 _____ F 11 _____

2 _____ 7 _____ 12 _____

3 _____ 8 _____ 13 _____

4 _____ 9 _____ 14 _____

5 _____ 10 _____ 15 _____

Number Correct [ ]

A Bear's Life

by T. E. Owens

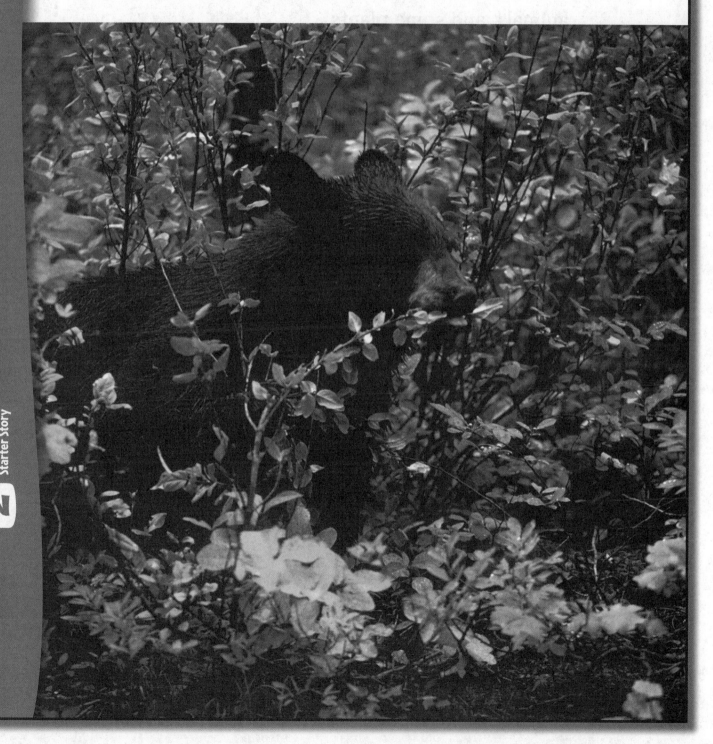

It's summer. You are playing ball. The black bear is looking for food.

It's winter. You are building snow castles. What is the black bear doing? It's sleeping.

That's a bear's life.

In summer it looks for food. It eats fish, small animals, and some plants.

When the leaves fall, there is more food. The bear eats fruit and nuts. It gets fat. The fat will come in handy when winter comes.

Then the bear makes its winter home. It digs a big hole under a tree. It goes inside to sleep. It doesn't need food then. It uses its fat to keep warm.

When spring comes, the bear leaves the hole. Summer is coming again!

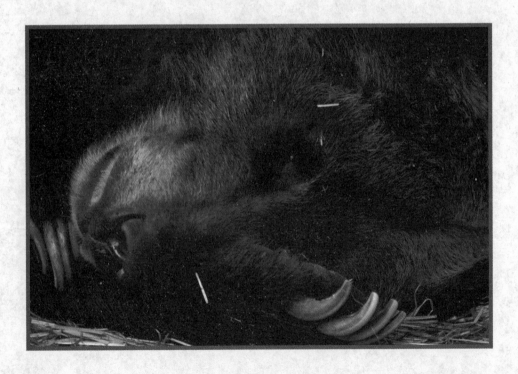

A Read each question. Write *a* or *b*.

1 What is this story about?
   a What black bears do in summer and winter
   b The games children play in summer and winter

2 How long does a bear sleep?
   a A bear sleeps all winter long.
   b A bear sleeps all summer long.

3 Why does a bear eat so much in the summer?
   a Because there isn't much food, and it is always hungry
   b Because it needs to be fat when winter comes

4 Why can a bear stay in a hole all winter long?
   a Because it takes fish and nuts into its hole
   b Because its fat makes it full and warm

5 What will a bear most likely do when it leaves its hole in the spring?
   a It will go to sleep.
   b It will look for food.

B b + at = bat

Look at each row of letters. Add one letter or group of letters from each row to *at* to make a word. Write the word.

1	gr, m, tr
2	th, cr, cl
3	q, f, d
4	z, g, s
5	c, j, l

+ at

C Read the words you wrote. Which one best fits in each sentence? Write the word.

6 The bear _____ down next to its hole.

7 A _____ doesn't sleep as long as a bear does.

8 The bear eats all the food _____ it can find.

9 It needs to get _____ before winter comes.

10 The bear sleeps on a _____ of dry leaves.

D Read each sentence. If the sentence tells why a bear sleeps in its hole all winter, write *Yes.* If it does not tell why a bear sleeps in its hole all winter, write *No.*

1 A bear digs a hole under a tree.

2 There is not much food for a bear when it snows.

3 A bear likes fish.

4 A hole helps a bear stay warm.

5 A bear looks for fruit and nuts.

Starter Story Record Page

Name _____   Date _____

Power Builder Color _____   Power Builder Number _____

A Comprehension

1 _____   2 _____   3 _____   4 _____   5 _____

Number Correct [ ]

B, C Learn about Words

1 _____   6 _____

2 _____   7 _____

3 _____   8 _____

4 _____   9 _____

5 _____   10 _____

Number Correct [ ]

Think about It

D 1 _____   **E** 6 _____   **F** 11 _____

2 _____   7 _____   12 _____

3 _____   8 _____   13 _____

4 _____   9 _____   14 _____

5 _____   10 _____   15 _____

Number Correct [ ]

Running

by Annie DeCaprio

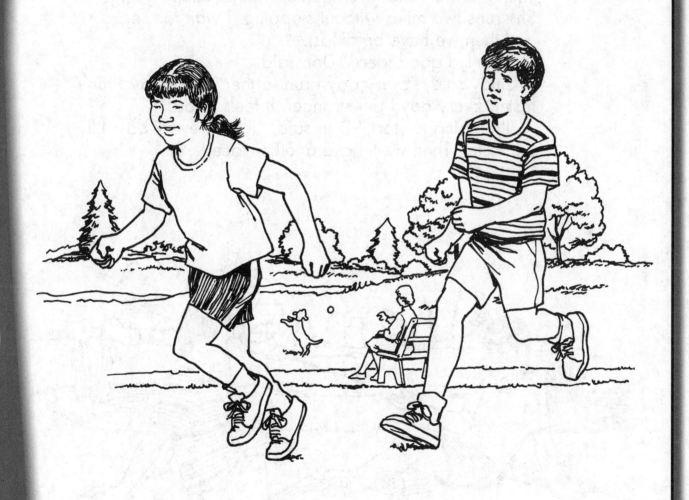

Cindy and Don ran a race. Cindy came in first.

"I'm bigger," Don said, "so why did you win? How did you run so fast?"

"I run every day," Cindy said. "I run with my mother. We go out before breakfast. We run around the park."

"Can you keep up with your mother?" Don asked.

"Yes," Cindy said. "But I don't run as far. I get tired. Then I turn around. I run home. Mother keeps going. She runs two miles without stopping. I wait for her, and then we have breakfast."

"That's a good idea," Don said.

Cindy said, "Every day I run farther. Every day I run faster. Every day I get stronger. It feels good."

"I'm going to start," Don said. "I'll run every day. I'll get faster. Then we'll have another race."

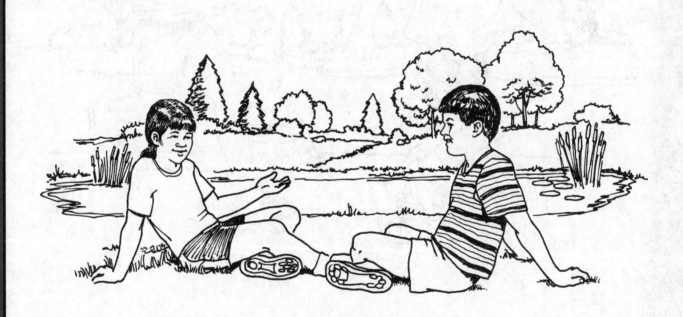

A Read each question. Write *a* or *b*.

1 What did Don find out in this story?
  a That growing bigger will make him a better runner
  b That running every day will make him a better runner

2 Why did Cindy win the race?
  a Because she was older than Don
  b Because she ran every day

3 Why does Cindy always turn around before her mother?
  a Because Cindy's mother is stronger than she is
  b Because Cindy wants to eat her breakfast alone

4 What does running every day do for Cindy?
  a It makes her strong.
  b It makes her big.

5 What did Don think after he talked to Cindy?
  a That he would work hard to be a better runner
  b That he didn't want to be a runner after all

LEARN ABOUT WORDS

B p + **ay** = **pay**

Look at each row of letters. Add one letter or group of letters from each row to *ay* to make a word. Write the word.

1 q, d, t
2 st, sr, gl
3 sm, sr, pl + **ay**
4 v, w, c
5 z, x, m

C Read the words you wrote. Which one best fits in each sentence? Write the word.

   6 Cindy likes to run and _____ games.
   7 She runs this _____ every day.
   8 Don and Cindy _____ have another race.
   9 Cindy does not _____ home when her mother runs.
   10 They run every _____ of the week.

Think about It

D Word pictures help you see things more clearly. They tell you more about a story. Choose the sentence that gives a better picture. Write *a* or *b*.

   1 a Don is much bigger than Cindy.
      b Don is two inches taller than Cindy.

   2 a Cindy and her mother run many places.
      b Cindy and her mother run by the park and the school.

   3 a They have toast and milk after they run.
      b They have some breakfast after they run.

   4 a Don wears his play clothes to the park.
      b Don wears shorts and running shoes to the park.

   5 a Cindy can run like the wind.
      b Cindy can run very fast.

Starter Story Record Page

Name _____ Date _____

Power Builder Color _____ Power Builder Number _____

A Comprehension

1 _____ 2 _____ 3 _____ 4 _____ 5 _____

Number Correct ☐

B, C Learn about Words

1 _____ 6 _____

2 _____ 7 _____

3 _____ 8 _____

4 _____ 9 _____

5 _____ 10 _____

Number Correct ☐

Think about It

D 1 _____ **E** 6 _____ **F** 11 _____

2 _____ 7 _____ 12 _____

3 _____ 8 _____ 13 _____

4 _____ 9 _____ 14 _____

5 _____ 10 _____ 15 _____

Number Correct ☐

A Funny Way to Become Famous

by John Savage

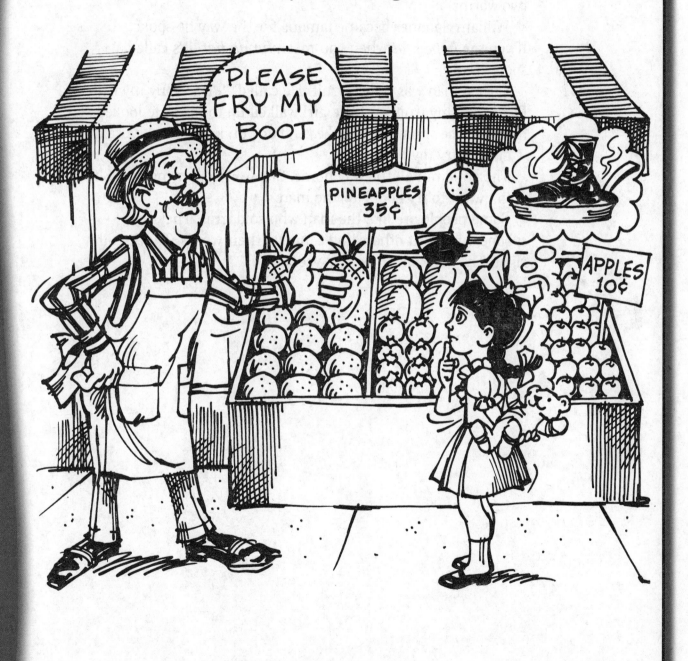

Once there was a man named William A. Spooner. He was a teacher.

When he spoke, he mixed up his words. He would say the first part of one word. Then he would add the last part of another word to it.

Once he scolded a student for loafing. He meant to say, "You have wasted two terms." But he said, "You have tasted two worms."

William Spooner became famous for the way he spoke. If you say *honey fat* when you mean *funny hat,* it's called a spoonerism.

Once a man was selling fruit. He called, "Please buy my fruit! Please buy my fruit!" A little girl walked up to him. He looked at her. Then he smiled and spoke. And do you know what he said?

"Please fry my boot!"

The child ran all the way home. She wanted her mother. She didn't want to fry boots for the man.

Some people are like the man who sold fruit. They say spoonerisms. But others don't mix up their words. They're all right. They talk like moo and yee.

A Choose the best ending for each sentence. Write *a* or *b*.

1 This story is about
 a how a fruit seller became famous.
 b how mixed-up words got a name.

2 A *spoonerism* is
 a a mixed-up way of saying things.
 b one of William Spooner's students.

3 If William Spooner were your teacher,
 a you might be mixed up sometimes.
 b you might have to taste worms.

4 When people use spoonerisms, they
 a are trying to be funny.
 b mean to say something else.

5 In the last line of this story, *moo and yee* really means
 a mine and yours.
 b you and me.

LEARN ABOUT WORDS

B Words change spelling when they mean more than one.

one book ⟶ two book**s**

Write each word below so that it means more than one.

1 Student
2 Word
3 Worm
4 Spoonerism
5 Mother

C Read the new words you wrote. Which word best fits in each sentence? Write the word.

6 William Spooner often said _____ in a funny way.
7 He said _____ when he meant to say *terms*.
8 Then all his _____ laughed.
9 They ran home to tell their _____ about him.
10 That is why mixed-up words are called _____ today.

THINK ABOUT IT

D Read each story. Write *a* or *b* to answer each question.

A little girl walked up to a man who was selling fruit. She wanted an apple. She took out some money.

1 What did the man do next?
  a Told the girl to go home
  b Sold the girl an apple

2 What did the girl do next?
  a Paid for the apple
  b Put her money away

3 How did you know what the man and the girl did?
  a The man was selling fruit. The girl had money to buy an apple.
  b The man didn't have any fruit. The girl didn't like apples.

Mr. Spooner handed each of his students a test. He told them to pick up their pencils and begin.

4 What did the students do next?
  a Took the test
  b Ate their lunches

5 How did you know what the students did?
  a They were hungry.
  b Mr. Spooner told them to begin.

E Read each set of words. Write the word that comes first in alphabetical order.

6	want	walked	way
7	soon	some	sold
8	who	what	when
9	fry	fruit	friend
10	said	say	same

Starter Story Record Page

Name _____ Date _____

Power Builder Color _____ Power Builder Number _____

A Comprehension

1 _____ 2 _____ 3 _____ 4 _____ 5 _____

Number Correct [   ]

B, C Learn about Words

1 _____ 6 _____

2 _____ 7 _____

3 _____ 8 _____

4 _____ 9 _____

5 _____ 10 _____

Number Correct [   ]

Think about It

D 1 _____ **E** 6 _____ **F** 11 _____

2 _____ 7 _____ 12 _____

3 _____ 8 _____ 13 _____

4 _____ 9 _____ 14 _____

5 _____ 10 _____ 15 _____

Number Correct [   ]

Room for One More?

by Gerry Armstrong

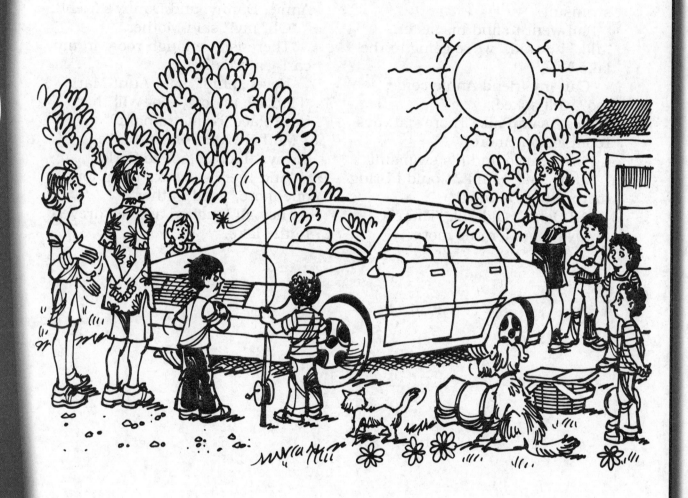

1   Father said, "It's a hot day. Let's go to the lake."

2   "Oh, good!" Mother said. "Call the children, dear."

3   Father went to call the children.

4   Mother said to herself, "Let's see, there's Jill and Phil and Father and me. I'll invite Aunt Mary, too. There's always room for one more."

5 Father said, "Phil, let's go to the lake."

6 Phil said, "Harry and I are playing. Could he come, too?"

7 "Yes," said Father. "There's always room for one more. Tell your sister that we're going."

8 Harry went home for his swimsuit.

9 Phil went to find his sister. "Jill," he said, "we're going to the lake."

10 "Can my friend Annie come, too?" Jill asked.

11 "Yes," said Phil. "There's always room for one more."

12 Phil went to find his swimsuit.

13 Annie said to Jill, "Could I bring my brother Danny?"

14 "All right," said Jill. "There's always room for one more."

15 Annie went home for her swimsuit and her brother. Danny wanted to bring a friend. "Oh, well," said Annie, "there's always room for one more."

16 They met by the car. There were Father and Mother; Jill and Phil; Aunt Mary and Harry. There were Annie, Danny, and Danny's friend.

17 "Oh, my!" said Mother.

18 "There isn't enough room in my car!" said Father.

19 "Never mind," said Aunt Mary. "I'll drive my car, too. Will there be a place for me to park?"

20 Mother said, "Oh, yes. We always find a place to park."

21 "And there's always room for one more," said Father.

22 They all laughed as they drove to the lake.

COMPREHENSION

A Choose the best ending for each sentence. Write *a* or *b*.

1 This story shows that
   a a big family can go everywhere together.
   b a little trouble doesn't have to stop everyone's fun.

2 Lots of people were going to the lake because
   a each one asked someone else to come.
   b Mother was having a big picnic.

3 Everyone thought there would be room for one more because
   a Mother and Father had a very large car.
   b no one knew how many people were coming.

4 When Aunt Mary said she would drive her car, too,
   a everyone got to go to the lake.
   b there still wasn't room for everyone.

5 The funny part of this story is
   a there really *was* room for one more.
   b everyone laughed as they drove to the lake.

LEARN ABOUT WORDS

B Often you can find out the meaning of a word by seeing how it is used in a story. The other words in the story give you clues.

Find the word in the story that best fits each meaning. (A paragraph number tells you where to look.) Write the word.

1 ask (4)
2 space (4)
3 look for and discover (9)
4 came together (16)
5 leave a car for a time (19)

C Read the words you wrote. Which one best fits in each sentence? Write the word.

6 Father said Phil could _____ Harry.
7 He told them to go and _____ their swimsuits.
8 There wasn't _____ for everybody in one car.
9 Aunt Mary had to _____ her car far away.
10 Aunt Mary _____ Mother and Father by the lake.

D The **bird's song** was as **sweet** as **honey.**

This sentence helps you understand how sweet the bird's song was. The phrase "as sweet as honey" is a **figure of speech.** It is a different way of saying that the bird's song was very lovely.

Choose the word from the first two sentences that best fits in the blank. Write the word.

1 An oven is hot. Ice is cold. It was as _____ as an oven that day.

2 A rabbit is fast. A turtle is slow. Father's car was as slow as a _____.

3 A lion is loud. A mouse is quiet. Jill was as quiet as a _____ at the lake.

4 A breeze is cool. Toast is warm. The water in the lake was as _____ as a breeze.

5 Coal is black. Snow is white. Aunt Mary's hair was as _____ as snow.

E sun + **light** = **sunlight**

The word *sunlight* means "the light of the sun." *Sunlight* is a **compound word.** A compound word is made by putting two or more words together.

Look at the two words in **bold type.** Put the two words together to complete the second sentence. Write the compound word.

6 Jill's **friend** was a **girl.** Jill invited her _____ to come.

7 Annie brought a **suit** to **swim** in. Her _____ was red.

8 Mother's **glasses** kept the **sun** out of her eyes. She wore a pair of _____.

9 Father's **boat** had a **house** on it. Everybody went for a ride on Father's _____.

10 The **fish** Phil caught looked like a **cat.** He was proud of his _____.

Starter Story Record Page

Name _____ Date _____

Power Builder Color _____ Power Builder Number _____

A Comprehension

1 _____ 2 _____ 3 _____ 4 _____ 5 _____

Number Correct [　　]

B, C Learn about Words

1 _____   6 _____

2 _____   7 _____

3 _____   8 _____

4 _____   9 _____

5 _____   10 _____

Number Correct [　　]

Think about It

D 1 _____ **E** 6 _____ **F** 11 _____

2 _____   7 _____   12 _____

3 _____   8 _____   13 _____

4 _____   9 _____   14 _____

5 _____   10 _____   15 _____

Number Correct [　　]

Starter Story

Mr. Dawson Has Cold Feet

by R. O. Work

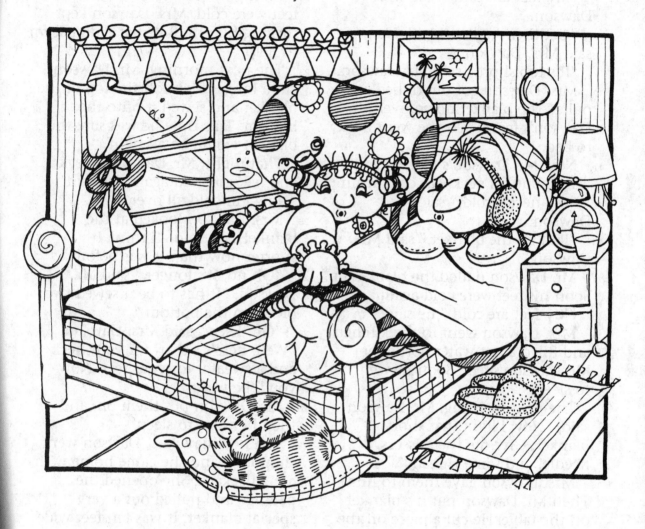

1   One night, Mr. Dawson said to his wife, "Marjorie, it's cold outside. Let's get out an extra blanket."

2   "All right, Donald," said Mrs. Dawson. "The blankets are in the cupboard. Let's get one now."

3   They went to the cupboard and got an old blanket. Then they went to bed.

4   "Marjorie," said Mr. Dawson, "I think this blanket shrank. I don't think it will keep me warm."

Adapted from *Mr. Dawson Had a Farm* by R. O. Work, copyright 1951, by the Bobbs-Merrill Company, Inc., reprinted by permission of the publishers and Betty J. Russell. Efforts to contact the owner of this copyrighted selection have not been successful. SRA will be glad to hear from the owner and to make appropriate permission arrangements.

5 "It will," said Mrs. Dawson.

6 Mr. Dawson closed his eyes. But he felt cold air around his neck. He pulled the blanket up higher.

7 "My feet are cold," said Mr. Dawson.

8 "Get them under the blanket," said Mrs. Dawson.

9 "It's too short," said Mr. Dawson.

10 Mrs. Dawson got out of bed and pulled the blanket down over Mr. Dawson's feet. Then she went back to bed.

11 Now Mr. Dawson's feet were warm. But his neck was cold again.

12 "My neck's cold," said Mr. Dawson.

13 "Pull up the blanket," said Mrs. Dawson.

14 Mr. Dawson pulled the blanket up. Soon his feet were cold again.

15 "My feet are cold," he said.

16 Mrs. Dawson went to the kitchen and filled a hot-water bottle for Mr. Dawson's feet. Soon he went to sleep.

17 The next morning, Mr. Dawson said, "Now I'll fix that short blanket. Give me the scissors, a needle, and some thread."

18 Mrs. Dawson gave them to him. Then Mr. Dawson put his blanket on the table. He cut a piece off the top of the blanket and sewed it onto the bottom.

19 Mr. Dawson went to bed early that night. Soon he felt the cold air on his neck. So he pulled the blanket up higher. Then his feet were cold.

20 "My feet are cold," Mr. Dawson said.

21 "Oh, not again!" said Mrs. Dawson.

22 All night, Mr. Dawson's neck and feet were cold. Mrs. Dawson kept tucking him in. But that didn't seem to help.

23 The next morning, Mr. Dawson cut a longer piece off the top of the blanket and sewed it onto the bottom. This time he was sure the blanket would be all right.

24 That night, Mr. Dawson's neck and feet got cold again. He said, "Now I'm cold all over."

25 Mrs. Dawson looked at the blanket. She said, "I think it's shorter now than it was before."

26 "Oh no, it's longer," said Mr. Dawson. "It has to be. I sewed two pieces to the bottom."

27 "Oh, I see," said Mrs. Dawson. "Well, here's a scarf for your neck and a sweater for your feet. Now you'll be warm."

28 Mr. Dawson put them on, and then he went to sleep.

29 The next day, Mrs. Dawson went shopping, and she came home with a big package. She opened the package and pulled out a very special blanket. It was ten feet wide and fifteen feet long.

30 "Oh, Marjorie," said Mr. Dawson, "that's a fine blanket. Now we both can get some sleep."

A Choose the best ending for each sentence. Write *a, b,* or *c.*

1 The joke in this story is that
 a Mr. and Mrs. Dawson kept blankets in a cupboard.
 b Mrs. Dawson got Mr. Dawson a sweater for his feet.
 c Mr. Dawson's sewing didn't really make the blanket longer.

2 Mr. Dawson couldn't sleep at night because
 a he was cold.
 b his bed was hard.
 c he wasn't tired.

3 Mr. Dawson *tried* to fix his problem by
 a making a new blanket.
 b making his blanket longer.
 c sewing a scarf to his blanket.

4 After Mr. Dawson cut and sewed his blanket, it was
 a shorter than before.
 b longer than before.
 c warmer than before.

5 Mr. Dawson finally got a good night's sleep because
 a Mrs. Dawson bought him a very big blanket.
 b Mr. Dawson sewed another piece on his old blanket.
 c the old blanket was finally big enough.

LEARN ABOUT WORDS

B Often you can find out the meaning of a word by seeing how it is used in a story. The other words in the story give you clues.

Find the word in the story that best fits each meaning. (A paragraph number tells you where to look.) Write the word.

1 warm covering for a bed (1)
2 place for keeping things (2)
3 became smaller when washed (4)
4 tool for cutting (17)
5 stitched (18)
6 cloth worn about the neck (27)
7 bundle; box with things in it (29)
8 unusual; not ordinary (29)

C A word may have more than one meaning. Its meaning will depend on how it is used.

My dad is a football *fan.*
He keeps cool with an electric *fan.*

Look at each word in **bold type** below. Note the paragraph number. Look back at the paragraph. Which meaning does the word have there? Write *a* or *b.*

→

9 **top** (18)
  a a toy that spins
  b upper end or part

10 **feet** (29)
  a units of measure
  b body parts below the ankles

THINK ABOUT IT

D A story has a beginning, a middle, and an end. A story has a problem. A story is about how someone tries to solve the problem.

Parts of a Story

Beginning tells
• Who
• Where
• The problem
Middle tells
• How someone tries to solve the problem
End tells
• How the problem is solved

Read each sentence. Does it tell about the beginning, the middle, or the end of the story? Write *beginning, middle,* or *end*.

1 Mr. Dawson tried to make the blanket longer.
2 Mrs. Dawson gave Mr. Dawson a sweater and a scarf.
3 The old blanket did not keep Mr. Dawson warm.
4 Mrs. Dawson bought a new blanket.
5 The weather got cold outside.

E Some contractions are made by putting a verb and *not* together.

wasn't is made from *was not*

Other contractions are made by putting a pronoun and a verb together.

that's is made from *that is*

we'll is made from *we will*

Read each sentence. Which two words make up each underlined contraction? Write the two words.

6 Mr. Dawson didn't understand.
7 He couldn't get warm.
8 Mrs. Dawson said, "Don't worry."
9 "Here's a new blanket," she said.
10 "Now I'll be happy!" Mr. Dawson said.

Starter Story Record Page

Name _____ Date _____

Power Builder Color _____ Power Builder Number _____

A Comprehension

1 _____ 2 _____ 3 _____ 4 _____ 5 _____

Number Correct [ ]

B, C Learn about Words

1 _____ 6 _____

2 _____ 7 _____

3 _____ 8 _____

4 _____ 9 _____

5 _____ 10 _____

Number Correct [ ]

Think about It

D 1 _____ **E** 6 _____ **F** 11 _____

2 _____ 7 _____ 12 _____

3 _____ 8 _____ 13 _____

4 _____ 9 _____ 14 _____

5 _____ 10 _____ 15 _____

Number Correct [ ]

Get Ready to Read . . .

When you read a story, you read sentences that belong together. They all help to tell about one **main idea.** The main idea is what the story is mostly about. Clues about the main idea will help you understand what you read. Here are some things to look for.

What Do You See?

You can use your eyes to get clues about the main idea of a story.

● **Look at the picture.**

● **Read the title.**

● **Read the first sentence.**

● **Read the last paragraph.**

All these clues will help you find the story's main idea.

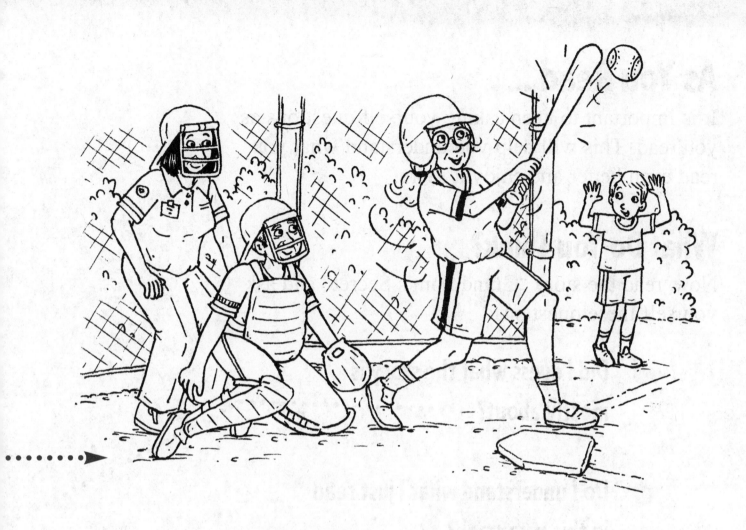

Grandmom's Secret

"Where is Grandmom going?" David asked. "She has a big bag and a softball bat."

"I don't know, David," Mom answered. "It's a secret. Grandpa says she goes out every Saturday."

Later, David went to the park. When he got there, he saw some grown-ups playing softball. Suddenly, the batter hit the ball. David was surprised. The batter was Grandmom!

As You Read . . .

It is important to keep asking yourself questions as you read. This will help you understand what you read even better and enjoy it more.

What Do You Think?

Now, read the story "Grandmom's Secret" and ask yourself these questions:

- **Did I guess what the story is mostly about?**

- **Do I understand what I just read in this paragraph?**

- **What did I learn from this story?**

These questions will help you get the most out of what you read.

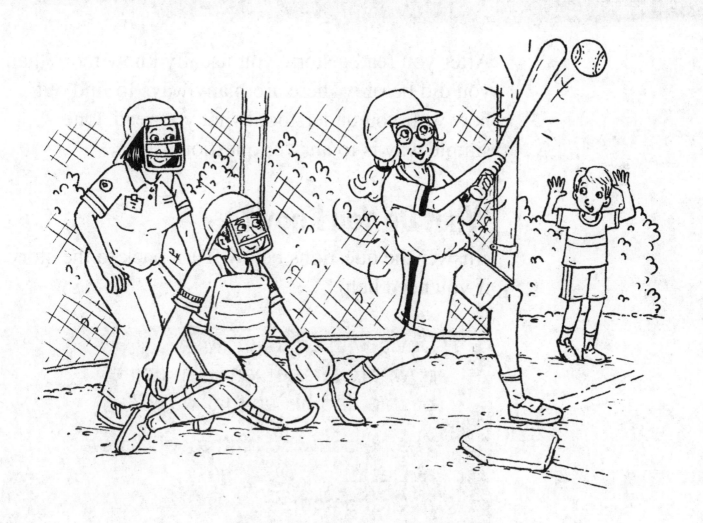

Grandmom's Secret

"Where is Grandmom going?" David asked. "She has a big bag and a softball bat."

"I don't know, David," Mom answered. "It's a secret. Grandpa says she goes out every Saturday."

Later, David went to the park. When he got there, he saw some grown-ups playing softball. Suddenly, the batter hit the ball. David was surprised. The batter was Grandmom!

After You Read . . .

After you read a story, you usually know more than you did before. There are many ways to find out how well you understood what you read. One simple way is to answer questions.

What Do You Know?

Answer the questions below. Turn back to the story if you need help.

1 David wanted to know
  a where Grandmom was going.
  b who had his softball bat.

2 The person who hit the softball was
  a David.
  b Grandmom.

3 The main idea is that
  a David's secret was that he visits Grandmom.
  b Grandmom's secret was that she plays softball.

4 Another good title for this story is
  a David's Softball Game.
  b Grandmom Plays Softball.

Go to page 128 in this book to check your answers.

Keep in Mind . . .

Before You Read

Use your eyes to get clues about the main idea:

- Look at the picture.

- Read the title.

- Read the first sentence.

- Read the last paragraph.

As You Read

Ask yourself these questions as you read to make sure you understand:

- Did I guess what the story is mostly about?

- Do I understand what I just read?

- What did I learn from this story?

Record Page

Name _____   Date _____

Power Builder Color _____   Power Builder Number _____

A Comprehension

1 _____   2 _____   3 _____   4 _____   5 _____

Number Correct [   ]

B, C Learn about Words

1 _____   6 _____

2 _____   7 _____

3 _____   8 _____

4 _____   9 _____

5 _____   10 _____

Number Correct [   ]

Think about It

D1 _____   E6 _____   F11 _____

2 _____   7 _____   12 _____

3 _____   8 _____   13 _____

4 _____   9 _____   14 _____

5 _____   10 _____   15 _____

Number Correct [   ]

Record Page

Name _____ Date _____

Power Builder Color _____ Power Builder Number _____

A Comprehension

1 _____ 2 _____ 3 _____ 4 _____ 5 _____

Number Correct [   ]

B, C Learn about Words

1 _____ 6 _____

2 _____ 7 _____

3 _____ 8 _____

4 _____ 9 _____

5 _____ 10 _____

Number Correct [   ]

Think about It

D 1 _____ E 6 _____ F 11 _____

2 _____ 7 _____ 12 _____

3 _____ 8 _____ 13 _____

4 _____ 9 _____ 14 _____

5 _____ 10 _____ 15 _____

Number Correct [   ]

Record Page

Name _____   Date _____

Power Builder Color _____   Power Builder Number _____

A Comprehension

1 _____ 2 _____ 3 _____ 4 _____ 5 _____

Number Correct [____]

B, C Learn about Words

1 _____   6 _____

2 _____   7 _____

3 _____   8 _____

4 _____   9 _____

5 _____   10 _____

Number Correct [____]

Think about It

D 1 _____   **E** 6 _____   **F** 11 _____

2 _____   7 _____   12 _____

3 _____   8 _____   13 _____

4 _____   9 _____   14 _____

5 _____   10 _____   15 _____

Number Correct [____]

Record Page

Name _____ Date _____

Power Builder Color _____ Power Builder Number _____

A Comprehension

1 _____ 2 _____ 3 _____ 4 _____ 5 _____

Number Correct [   ]

B, C Learn about Words

1 _____   6 _____

2 _____   7 _____

3 _____   8 _____

4 _____   9 _____

5 _____   10 _____

Number Correct [   ]

Think about It

D 1 _____   **E** 6 _____   **F** 11 _____

2 _____   7 _____   12 _____

3 _____   8 _____   13 _____

4 _____   9 _____   14 _____

5 _____   10 _____   15 _____

Number Correct [   ]

Record Page

Name _____ Date _____

Power Builder Color _____ Power Builder Number _____

A Comprehension

1 _____ 2 _____ 3 _____ 4 _____ 5 _____

Number Correct [ ]

B, C Learn about Words

1 _____ 6 _____

2 _____ 7 _____

3 _____ 8 _____

4 _____ 9 _____

5 _____ 10 _____

Number Correct [ ]

Think about It

D 1 _____ **E** 6 _____ **F** 11 _____

2 _____ 7 _____ 12 _____

3 _____ 8 _____ 13 _____

4 _____ 9 _____ 14 _____

5 _____ 10 _____ 15 _____

Number Correct [ ]

Record Page

Name _____ Date _____

Power Builder Color _____ Power Builder Number _____

A Comprehension

1 _____ 2 _____ 3 _____ 4 _____ 5 _____

Number Correct [＿＿]

B, C Learn about Words

1 _____ 6 _____

2 _____ 7 _____

3 _____ 8 _____

4 _____ 9 _____

5 _____ 10 _____

Number Correct [＿＿]

Think about It

D 1 _____ **E** 6 _____ **F** 11 _____

2 _____ 7 _____ 12 _____

3 _____ 8 _____ 13 _____

4 _____ 9 _____ 14 _____

5 _____ 10 _____ 15 _____

Number Correct [＿＿]

Record Page

Name _____ Date _____

Power Builder Color _____ Power Builder Number _____

A Comprehension

1 _____ 2 _____ 3 _____ 4 _____ 5 _____

Number Correct [ ]

B, C Learn about Words

1 _____ 6 _____

2 _____ 7 _____

3 _____ 8 _____

4 _____ 9 _____

5 _____ 10 _____

Number Correct [ ]

Think about It

D 1 _____ **E** 6 _____ **F** 11 _____

2 _____ 7 _____ 12 _____

3 _____ 8 _____ 13 _____

4 _____ 9 _____ 14 _____

5 _____ 10 _____ 15 _____

Number Correct [ ]

Record Page

Name _____ Date _____

Power Builder Color _____ Power Builder Number _____

A Comprehension

1 _____ 2 _____ 3 _____ 4 _____ 5 _____

Number Correct [   ]

B, C Learn about Words

1 _____ 6 _____

2 _____ 7 _____

3 _____ 8 _____

4 _____ 9 _____

5 _____ 10 _____

Number Correct [   ]

Think about It

D 1 _____ **E** 6 _____ **F** 11 _____

2 _____ 7 _____ 12 _____

3 _____ 8 _____ 13 _____

4 _____ 9 _____ 14 _____

5 _____ 10 _____ 15 _____

Number Correct [   ]

Record Page

Name _____ Date _____

Power Builder Color _____ Power Builder Number _____

A Comprehension

1 _____ 2 _____ 3 _____ 4 _____ 5 _____

Number Correct [   ]

B, C Learn about Words

1 _____   6 _____

2 _____   7 _____

3 _____   8 _____

4 _____   9 _____

5 _____   10 _____

Number Correct [   ]

Think about It

D 1 _____ **E** 6 _____ **F** 11 _____

2 _____   7 _____   12 _____

3 _____   8 _____   13 _____

4 _____   9 _____   14 _____

5 _____   10 _____   15 _____

Number Correct [   ]

Record Page

Name _____ Date _____

Power Builder Color _____ Power Builder Number _____

A Comprehension

1 _____ 2 _____ 3 _____ 4 _____ 5 _____

Number Correct [ ]

B, C Learn about Words

1 _____   6 _____

2 _____   7 _____

3 _____   8 _____

4 _____   9 _____

5 _____   10 _____

Number Correct [ ]

Think about It

D 1 _____   **E** 6 _____   **F** 11 _____

2 _____   7 _____   12 _____

3 _____   8 _____   13 _____

4 _____   9 _____   14 _____

5 _____   10 _____   15 _____

Number Correct [ ]

Record Page

Name _____ Date _____

Power Builder Color _____ Power Builder Number _____

A Comprehension

1 _____ 2 _____ 3 _____ 4 _____ 5 _____

Number Correct [   ]

B, C Learn about Words

1 _____ 6 _____

2 _____ 7 _____

3 _____ 8 _____

4 _____ 9 _____

5 _____ 10 _____

Number Correct [   ]

Think about It

D 1 _____ **E** 6 _____ **F** 11 _____

2 _____ 7 _____ 12 _____

3 _____ 8 _____ 13 _____

4 _____ 9 _____ 14 _____

5 _____ 10 _____ 15 _____

Number Correct [   ]

Record Page

Name _____ Date _____

Power Builder Color _____ Power Builder Number _____

A Comprehension

1 _____ 2 _____ 3 _____ 4 _____ 5 _____

Number Correct [ ]

B, C Learn about Words

1 _____   6 _____

2 _____   7 _____

3 _____   8 _____

4 _____   9 _____

5 _____   10 _____

Number Correct [ ]

Think about It

D 1 _____   **E** 6 _____   **F** 11 _____

2 _____   7 _____   12 _____

3 _____   8 _____   13 _____

4 _____   9 _____   14 _____

5 _____   10 _____   15 _____

Number Correct [ ]

Record Page

Name _____ Date _____

Power Builder Color _____ Power Builder Number _____

A Comprehension

1 _____ 2 _____ 3 _____ 4 _____ 5 _____

Number Correct [   ]

B, C Learn about Words

1 _____   6 _____

2 _____   7 _____

3 _____   8 _____

4 _____   9 _____

5 _____   10 _____

Number Correct [   ]

Think about It

D 1 _____   **E** 6 _____   **F** 11 _____

2 _____   7 _____   12 _____

3 _____   8 _____   13 _____

4 _____   9 _____   14 _____

5 _____   10 _____   15 _____

Number Correct [   ]

Record Page

Name _____   Date _____

Power Builder Color _____   Power Builder Number _____

A Comprehension

1 _____ 2 _____ 3 _____ 4 _____ 5 _____

Number Correct [   ]

B, C Learn about Words

1 _____   6 _____

2 _____   7 _____

3 _____   8 _____

4 _____   9 _____

5 _____   10 _____

Number Correct [   ]

Think about It

D 1 _____ **E** 6 _____ **F** 11 _____

2 _____   7 _____   12 _____

3 _____   8 _____   13 _____

4 _____   9 _____   14 _____

5 _____   10 _____   15 _____

Number Correct [   ]

Record Page

Name _____ Date _____

Power Builder Color _____ Power Builder Number _____

A Comprehension

1 _____ 2 _____ 3 _____ 4 _____ 5 _____

Number Correct [ ]

B, C Learn about Words

1 _____ 6 _____

2 _____ 7 _____

3 _____ 8 _____

4 _____ 9 _____

5 _____ 10 _____

Number Correct [ ]

Think about It

D 1 _____ **E** 6 _____ **F** 11 _____

2 _____ 7 _____ 12 _____

3 _____ 8 _____ 13 _____

4 _____ 9 _____ 14 _____

5 _____ 10 _____ 15 _____

Number Correct [ ]

Record Page

Name _____ Date _____

Power Builder Color _____ Power Builder Number _____

A Comprehension

1 _____ 2 _____ 3 _____ 4 _____ 5 _____

Number Correct [ ]

B, C Learn about Words

1 _____ 6 _____

2 _____ 7 _____

3 _____ 8 _____

4 _____ 9 _____

5 _____ 10 _____

Number Correct [ ]

Think about It

D 1 _____   E 6 _____   F 11 _____

2 _____   7 _____   12 _____

3 _____   8 _____   13 _____

4 _____   9 _____   14 _____

5 _____   10 _____   15 _____

Number Correct [ ]

Record Page

Name _____ Date _____

Power Builder Color _____ Power Builder Number _____

A Comprehension

1 _____ 2 _____ 3 _____ 4 _____ 5 _____

Number Correct [   ]

B, C Learn about Words

1 _____   6 _____

2 _____   7 _____

3 _____   8 _____

4 _____   9 _____

5 _____   10 _____

Number Correct [   ]

Think about It

D 1 _____   **E** 6 _____   **F** 11 _____

2 _____   7 _____   12 _____

3 _____   8 _____   13 _____

4 _____   9 _____   14 _____

5 _____   10 _____   15 _____

Number Correct [   ]

Record Page

Name _____ Date _____

Power Builder Color _____ Power Builder Number _____

A Comprehension

1 _____ 2 _____ 3 _____ 4 _____ 5 _____

Number Correct [   ]

B, C Learn about Words

1 _____ 6 _____

2 _____ 7 _____

3 _____ 8 _____

4 _____ 9 _____

5 _____ 10 _____

Number Correct [   ]

Think about It

D 1 _____ **E** 6 _____ **F** 11 _____

2 _____ 7 _____ 12 _____

3 _____ 8 _____ 13 _____

4 _____ 9 _____ 14 _____

5 _____ 10 _____ 15 _____

Number Correct [   ]

Record Page

Name _____ Date _____

Power Builder Color _____ Power Builder Number _____

A Comprehension

1 _____ 2 _____ 3 _____ 4 _____ 5 _____

Number Correct [ ]

B, C Learn about Words

1 _____ 6 _____

2 _____ 7 _____

3 _____ 8 _____

4 _____ 9 _____

5 _____ 10 _____

Number Correct [ ]

Think about It

D 1 _____ **E** 6 _____ **F** 11 _____

2 _____ 7 _____ 12 _____

3 _____ 8 _____ 13 _____

4 _____ 9 _____ 14 _____

5 _____ 10 _____ 15 _____

Number Correct [ ]

Record Page

Name _____ Date _____

Power Builder Color _____ Power Builder Number _____

A Comprehension

1 _____ 2 _____ 3 _____ 4 _____ 5 _____

Number Correct ☐

B, C Learn about Words

1 _____ 6 _____

2 _____ 7 _____

3 _____ 8 _____

4 _____ 9 _____

5 _____ 10 _____

Number Correct ☐

Think about It

D 1 _____ **E** 6 _____ **F** 11 _____

2 _____ 7 _____ 12 _____

3 _____ 8 _____ 13 _____

4 _____ 9 _____ 14 _____

5 _____ 10 _____ 15 _____

Number Correct ☐

Record Page

Name _____ Date _____

Power Builder Color _____ Power Builder Number _____

A Comprehension

1 _____ 2 _____ 3 _____ 4 _____ 5 _____

Number Correct ☐

B, C Learn about Words

1 _____ 6 _____

2 _____ 7 _____

3 _____ 8 _____

4 _____ 9 _____

5 _____ 10 _____

Number Correct ☐

Think about It

D 1 _____ **E** 6 _____ **F** 11 _____

2 _____ 7 _____ 12 _____

3 _____ 8 _____ 13 _____

4 _____ 9 _____ 14 _____

5 _____ 10 _____ 15 _____

Number Correct ☐

Record Page

Name _____ Date _____

Power Builder Color _____ Power Builder Number _____

A Comprehension

1 _____ 2 _____ 3 _____ 4 _____ 5 _____

Number Correct [ ]

B, C Learn about Words

1 _____   6 _____

2 _____   7 _____

3 _____   8 _____

4 _____   9 _____

5 _____   10 _____

Number Correct [ ]

Think about It

D 1 _____   **E** 6 _____   **F** 11 _____

2 _____   7 _____   12 _____

3 _____   8 _____   13 _____

4 _____   9 _____   14 _____

5 _____   10 _____   15 _____

Number Correct [ ]

Record Page

Name _____ Date _____

Power Builder Color _____ Power Builder Number _____

A Comprehension

1 _____ 2 _____ 3 _____ 4 _____ 5 _____

Number Correct [   ]

B, C Learn about Words

1 _____   6 _____

2 _____   7 _____

3 _____   8 _____

4 _____   9 _____

5 _____   10 _____

Number Correct [   ]

Think about It

D 1 _____   **E** 6 _____   **F** 11 _____

2 _____   7 _____   12 _____

3 _____   8 _____   13 _____

4 _____   9 _____   14 _____

5 _____   10 _____   15 _____

Number Correct [   ]

Record Page

Name _____ Date _____

Power Builder Color _____ Power Builder Number _____

A Comprehension

1 _____ 2 _____ 3 _____ 4 _____ 5 _____

Number Correct [ ]

B, C Learn about Words

1 _____ 6 _____

2 _____ 7 _____

3 _____ 8 _____

4 _____ 9 _____

5 _____ 10 _____

Number Correct [ ]

Think about It

D 1 _____ **E** 6 _____ **F** 11 _____

2 _____ 7 _____ 12 _____

3 _____ 8 _____ 13 _____

4 _____ 9 _____ 14 _____

5 _____ 10 _____ 15 _____

Number Correct [ ]

Record Page

Name _____ Date _____

Power Builder Color _____ Power Builder Number _____

A Comprehension

1 _____ 2 _____ 3 _____ 4 _____ 5 _____

Number Correct [ ]

B, C Learn about Words

1 _____   6 _____

2 _____   7 _____

3 _____   8 _____

4 _____   9 _____

5 _____   10 _____

Number Correct [ ]

Think about It

D 1 _____   **E** 6 _____   **F** 11 _____

2 _____   7 _____   12 _____

3 _____   8 _____   13 _____

4 _____   9 _____   14 _____

5 _____   10 _____   15 _____

Number Correct [ ]

Record Page

Name _____ Date _____

Power Builder Color _____ Power Builder Number _____

A Comprehension

1 _____ 2 _____ 3 _____ 4 _____ 5 _____

Number Correct [   ]

B, C Learn about Words

1 _____   6 _____

2 _____   7 _____

3 _____   8 _____

4 _____   9 _____

5 _____   10 _____

Number Correct [   ]

Think about It

D 1 _____   **E** 6 _____   **F** 11 _____

2 _____   7 _____   12 _____

3 _____   8 _____   13 _____

4 _____   9 _____   14 _____

5 _____   10 _____   15 _____

Number Correct [   ]

Record Page

Name _____ Date _____

Power Builder Color _____ Power Builder Number _____

A Comprehension

1 _____ 2 _____ 3 _____ 4 _____ 5 _____

Number Correct [   ]

B, C Learn about Words

1 _____   6 _____

2 _____   7 _____

3 _____   8 _____

4 _____   9 _____

5 _____   10 _____

Number Correct [   ]

Think about It

D 1 _____   **E** 6 _____   **F** 11 _____

2 _____   7 _____   12 _____

3 _____   8 _____   13 _____

4 _____   9 _____   14 _____

5 _____   10 _____   15 _____

Number Correct [   ]

Record Page

Name _____ Date _____

Power Builder Color _____ Power Builder Number _____

A Comprehension

1 _____ 2 _____ 3 _____ 4 _____ 5 _____

Number Correct ☐

B, C Learn about Words

1 _____   6 _____

2 _____   7 _____

3 _____   8 _____

4 _____   9 _____

5 _____   10 _____

Number Correct ☐

Think about It

D 1 _____   **E** 6 _____   **F** 11 _____

2 _____   7 _____   12 _____

3 _____   8 _____   13 _____

4 _____   9 _____   14 _____

5 _____   10 _____   15 _____

Number Correct ☐

Record Page

Name _____ Date _____

Power Builder Color _____ Power Builder Number _____

A Comprehension

1 _____ 2 _____ 3 _____ 4 _____ 5 _____

Number Correct [   ]

B, C Learn about Words

1 _____ 6 _____

2 _____ 7 _____

3 _____ 8 _____

4 _____ 9 _____

5 _____ 10 _____

Number Correct [   ]

Think about It

D 1 _____ E 6 _____ F 11 _____

2 _____ 7 _____ 12 _____

3 _____ 8 _____ 13 _____

4 _____ 9 _____ 14 _____

5 _____ 10 _____ 15 _____

Number Correct [   ]

Record Page

Name _____ Date _____

Power Builder Color _____ Power Builder Number _____

A Comprehension

1 _____ 2 _____ 3 _____ 4 _____ 5 _____

Number Correct [ ]

B, C Learn about Words

1 _____ 6 _____

2 _____ 7 _____

3 _____ 8 _____

4 _____ 9 _____

5 _____ 10 _____

Number Correct [ ]

Think about It

D 1 _____ **E** 6 _____ **F** 11 _____

2 _____ 7 _____ 12 _____

3 _____ 8 _____ 13 _____

4 _____ 9 _____ 14 _____

5 _____ 10 _____ 15 _____

Number Correct [ ]

Record Page

Name _____ Date _____

Power Builder Color _____ Power Builder Number _____

A Comprehension

1 _____ 2 _____ 3 _____ 4 _____ 5 _____

Number Correct ☐

B, C Learn about Words

1 _____ 6 _____

2 _____ 7 _____

3 _____ 8 _____

4 _____ 9 _____

5 _____ 10 _____

Number Correct ☐

Think about It

D 1 _____ **E** 6 _____ **F** 11 _____

2 _____ 7 _____ 12 _____

3 _____ 8 _____ 13 _____

4 _____ 9 _____ 14 _____

5 _____ 10 _____ 15 _____

Number Correct ☐

Record Page

Name _____ Date _____

Power Builder Color _____ Power Builder Number _____

A Comprehension

1 _____ 2 _____ 3 _____ 4 _____ 5 _____

Number Correct [   ]

B, C Learn about Words

1 _____ 6 _____

2 _____ 7 _____

3 _____ 8 _____

4 _____ 9 _____

5 _____ 10 _____

Number Correct [   ]

Think about It

D 1 _____ **E** 6 _____ **F** 11 _____

2 _____ 7 _____ 12 _____

3 _____ 8 _____ 13 _____

4 _____ 9 _____ 14 _____

5 _____ 10 _____ 15 _____

Number Correct [   ]

Record Page

Name _____ Date _____

Power Builder Color _____ Power Builder Number _____

A Comprehension

1 _____ 2 _____ 3 _____ 4 _____ 5 _____

Number Correct [ ]

B, C Learn about Words

1 _____ 6 _____

2 _____ 7 _____

3 _____ 8 _____

4 _____ 9 _____

5 _____ 10 _____

Number Correct [ ]

Think about It

D 1 _____ **E** 6 _____ **F** 11 _____

2 _____ 7 _____ 12 _____

3 _____ 8 _____ 13 _____

4 _____ 9 _____ 14 _____

5 _____ 10 _____ 15 _____

Number Correct [ ]

Record Page

Name _____ Date _____

Power Builder Color _____ Power Builder Number _____

A Comprehension

1 _____ 2 _____ 3 _____ 4 _____ 5 _____

Number Correct ☐

B, C Learn about Words

1 _____   6 _____

2 _____   7 _____

3 _____   8 _____

4 _____   9 _____

5 _____   10 _____

Number Correct ☐

Think about It

D 1 _____   **E** 6 _____   **F** 11 _____

2 _____   7 _____   12 _____

3 _____   8 _____   13 _____

4 _____   9 _____   14 _____

5 _____   10 _____   15 _____

Number Correct ☐

Record Page

Name _____ Date _____

Power Builder Color _____ Power Builder Number _____

A Comprehension

1 _____ 2 _____ 3 _____ 4 _____ 5 _____

Number Correct [ ]

B, C Learn about Words

1 _____ 6 _____

2 _____ 7 _____

3 _____ 8 _____

4 _____ 9 _____

5 _____ 10 _____

Number Correct [ ]

Think about It

D 1 _____ **E** 6 _____ **F** 11 _____

2 _____ 7 _____ 12 _____

3 _____ 8 _____ 13 _____

4 _____ 9 _____ 14 _____

5 _____ 10 _____ 15 _____

Number Correct [ ]

Record Page

Name _____ Date _____

Power Builder Color _____ Power Builder Number _____

A Comprehension

1 _____ 2 _____ 3 _____ 4 _____ 5 _____

Number Correct ☐

B, C Learn about Words

1 _____   6 _____

2 _____   7 _____

3 _____   8 _____

4 _____   9 _____

5 _____   10 _____

Number Correct ☐

Think about It

D 1 _____   **E** 6 _____   **F** 11 _____

2 _____   7 _____   12 _____

3 _____   8 _____   13 _____

4 _____   9 _____   14 _____

5 _____   10 _____   15 _____

Number Correct ☐

Record Page

Name _____ Date _____

Power Builder Color _____ Power Builder Number _____

A Comprehension

1 _____ 2 _____ 3 _____ 4 _____ 5 _____

Number Correct [   ]

B, C Learn about Words

1 _____   6 _____

2 _____   7 _____

3 _____   8 _____

4 _____   9 _____

5 _____   10 _____

Number Correct [   ]

Think about It

D 1 _____ **E** 6 _____ **F** 11 _____

2 _____   7 _____   12 _____

3 _____   8 _____   13 _____

4 _____   9 _____   14 _____

5 _____   10 _____   15 _____

Number Correct [   ]

Record Page

Name _____ Date _____

Power Builder Color _____ Power Builder Number _____

A Comprehension

1 _____ 2 _____ 3 _____ 4 _____ 5 _____

Number Correct [   ]

B, C Learn about Words

1 _____ 6 _____

2 _____ 7 _____

3 _____ 8 _____

4 _____ 9 _____

5 _____ 10 _____

Number Correct [   ]

Think about It

D 1 _____ **E** 6 _____ **F** 11 _____

2 _____ 7 _____ 12 _____

3 _____ 8 _____ 13 _____

4 _____ 9 _____ 14 _____

5 _____ 10 _____ 15 _____

Number Correct [   ]

Record Page

Name _____   Date _____

Power Builder Color _____   Power Builder Number _____

A Comprehension

1 _____ 2 _____ 3 _____ 4 _____ 5 _____

Number Correct [　]

B, C Learn about Words

1 _____   6 _____

2 _____   7 _____

3 _____   8 _____

4 _____   9 _____

5 _____   10 _____

Number Correct [　]

Think about It

D 1 _____   **E** 6 _____   **F** 11 _____

2 _____   7 _____   12 _____

3 _____   8 _____   13 _____

4 _____   9 _____   14 _____

5 _____   10 _____   15 _____

Number Correct [　]

Record Page

Name _____   Date _____

Power Builder Color _____   Power Builder Number _____

A Comprehension

1 _____ 2 _____ 3 _____ 4 _____ 5 _____

Number Correct [ ]

B, C Learn about Words

1 _____   6 _____

2 _____   7 _____

3 _____   8 _____

4 _____   9 _____

5 _____   10 _____

Number Correct [ ]

Think about It

D 1 _____   **E** 6 _____   **F** 11 _____

2 _____   7 _____   12 _____

3 _____   8 _____   13 _____

4 _____   9 _____   14 _____

5 _____   10 _____   15 _____

Number Correct [ ]

Record Page

Name _____ Date _____

Power Builder Color _____ Power Builder Number _____

A Comprehension

1 _____ 2 _____ 3 _____ 4 _____ 5 _____

Number Correct [   ]

B, C Learn about Words

1 _____   6 _____

2 _____   7 _____

3 _____   8 _____

4 _____   9 _____

5 _____   10 _____

Number Correct [   ]

Think about It

D 1 _____   **E** 6 _____   **F** 11 _____

2 _____   7 _____   12 _____

3 _____   8 _____   13 _____

4 _____   9 _____   14 _____

5 _____   10 _____   15 _____

Number Correct [   ]

Record Page

Name _____ Date _____

Power Builder Color _____ Power Builder Number _____

A Comprehension

1 _____ 2 _____ 3 _____ 4 _____ 5 _____

Number Correct ☐

B, C Learn about Words

1 _____ 6 _____

2 _____ 7 _____

3 _____ 8 _____

4 _____ 9 _____

5 _____ 10 _____

Number Correct ☐

Think about It

D 1 _____ **E** 6 _____ **F** 11 _____

2 _____ 7 _____ 12 _____

3 _____ 8 _____ 13 _____

4 _____ 9 _____ 14 _____

5 _____ 10 _____ 15 _____

Number Correct ☐

Record Page

Name _____ Date _____

Power Builder Color _____ Power Builder Number _____

A Comprehension

1 _____ 2 _____ 3 _____ 4 _____ 5 _____

Number Correct [ ]

B, C Learn about Words

1 _____ 6 _____

2 _____ 7 _____

3 _____ 8 _____

4 _____ 9 _____

5 _____ 10 _____

Number Correct [ ]

Think about It

D 1 _____ **E** 6 _____ **F** 11 _____

2 _____ 7 _____ 12 _____

3 _____ 8 _____ 13 _____

4 _____ 9 _____ 14 _____

5 _____ 10 _____ 15 _____

Number Correct [ ]

Record Page

Name _____ Date _____

Power Builder Color _____ Power Builder Number _____

A Comprehension

1 _____ 2 _____ 3 _____ 4 _____ 5 _____

Number Correct ☐

B, C Learn about Words

1 _____ 6 _____

2 _____ 7 _____

3 _____ 8 _____

4 _____ 9 _____

5 _____ 10 _____

Number Correct ☐

Think about It

D1 _____ **E**6 _____ **F**11 _____

2 _____ 7 _____ 12 _____

3 _____ 8 _____ 13 _____

4 _____ 9 _____ 14 _____

5 _____ 10 _____ 15 _____

Number Correct ☐

Record Page

Name _____ Date _____

Power Builder Color _____ Power Builder Number _____

A Comprehension

1 _____ 2 _____ 3 _____ 4 _____ 5 _____

Number Correct [ ]

B, C Learn about Words

1 _____ 6 _____

2 _____ 7 _____

3 _____ 8 _____

4 _____ 9 _____

5 _____ 10 _____

Number Correct [ ]

Think about It

D 1 _____ **E** 6 _____ **F** 11 _____

2 _____ 7 _____ 12 _____

3 _____ 8 _____ 13 _____

4 _____ 9 _____ 14 _____

5 _____ 10 _____ 15 _____

Number Correct [ ]

Record Page

Name _____ Date _____

Power Builder Color _____ Power Builder Number _____

A Comprehension

1 _____ 2 _____ 3 _____ 4 _____ 5 _____

Number Correct [   ]

B, C Learn about Words

1 _____ 6 _____

2 _____ 7 _____

3 _____ 8 _____

4 _____ 9 _____

5 _____ 10 _____

Number Correct [   ]

Think about It

D 1 _____ **E** 6 _____ **F** 11 _____

2 _____ 7 _____ 12 _____

3 _____ 8 _____ 13 _____

4 _____ 9 _____ 14 _____

5 _____ 10 _____ 15 _____

Number Correct [   ]

Record Page

Name _____ Date _____

Power Builder Color _____ Power Builder Number _____

A Comprehension

1 _____ 2 _____ 3 _____ 4 _____ 5 _____

Number Correct [ ]

B, C Learn about Words

1 _____ 6 _____

2 _____ 7 _____

3 _____ 8 _____

4 _____ 9 _____

5 _____ 10 _____

Number Correct [ ]

Think about It

D 1 _____ **E** 6 _____ **F** 11 _____

2 _____ 7 _____ 12 _____

3 _____ 8 _____ 13 _____

4 _____ 9 _____ 14 _____

5 _____ 10 _____ 15 _____

Number Correct [ ]

Record Page

Name _____ Date _____

Power Builder Color _____ Power Builder Number _____

A Comprehension

1 _____ 2 _____ 3 _____ 4 _____ 5 _____

Number Correct [　　]

B, C Learn about Words

1 _____ 6 _____

2 _____ 7 _____

3 _____ 8 _____

4 _____ 9 _____

5 _____ 10 _____

Number Correct [　　]

Think about It

D 1 _____ **E** 6 _____ **F** 11 _____

2 _____ 7 _____ 12 _____

3 _____ 8 _____ 13 _____

4 _____ 9 _____ 14 _____

5 _____ 10 _____ 15 _____

Number Correct [　　]

Record Page

Name _____ Date _____

Power Builder Color _____ Power Builder Number _____

A Comprehension

1 _____ 2 _____ 3 _____ 4 _____ 5 _____

Number Correct [   ]

B, C Learn about Words

1 _____ 6 _____

2 _____ 7 _____

3 _____ 8 _____

4 _____ 9 _____

5 _____ 10 _____

Number Correct [   ]

Think about It

D 1 _____ E 6 _____ F 11 _____

2 _____ 7 _____ 12 _____

3 _____ 8 _____ 13 _____

4 _____ 9 _____ 14 _____

5 _____ 10 _____ 15 _____

Number Correct [   ]

Record Page

Name _____ Date _____

Power Builder Color _____ Power Builder Number _____

A Comprehension

1 _____ 2 _____ 3 _____ 4 _____ 5 _____

Number Correct [   ]

B, C Learn about Words

1 _____ 6 _____

2 _____ 7 _____

3 _____ 8 _____

4 _____ 9 _____

5 _____ 10 _____

Number Correct [   ]

Think about It

D 1 _____ **E** 6 _____ **F** 11 _____

2 _____ 7 _____ 12 _____

3 _____ 8 _____ 13 _____

4 _____ 9 _____ 14 _____

5 _____ 10 _____ 15 _____

Number Correct [   ]

Record Page

Name _____ Date _____

Power Builder Color _____ Power Builder Number _____

A Comprehension

1 _____ 2 _____ 3 _____ 4 _____ 5 _____

Number Correct ☐

B, C Learn about Words

1 _____ 6 _____

2 _____ 7 _____

3 _____ 8 _____

4 _____ 9 _____

5 _____ 10 _____

Number Correct ☐

Think about It

D 1 _____ **E** 6 _____ **F** 11 _____

2 _____ 7 _____ 12 _____

3 _____ 8 _____ 13 _____

4 _____ 9 _____ 14 _____

5 _____ 10 _____ 15 _____

Number Correct ☐

Record Page

Name _____ Date _____

Power Builder Color _____ Power Builder Number _____

A Comprehension

1 _____ 2 _____ 3 _____ 4 _____ 5 _____

Number Correct [   ]

B, C Learn about Words

1 _____ 6 _____

2 _____ 7 _____

3 _____ 8 _____

4 _____ 9 _____

5 _____ 10 _____

Number Correct [   ]

Think about It

D 1 _____ **E** 6 _____ **F** 11 _____

2 _____ 7 _____ 12 _____

3 _____ 8 _____ 13 _____

4 _____ 9 _____ 14 _____

5 _____ 10 _____ 15 _____

Number Correct [   ]

Record Page

Name _____ Date _____

Power Builder Color _____ Power Builder Number _____

A Comprehension

1 _____ 2 _____ 3 _____ 4 _____ 5 _____

Number Correct [ ]

B, C Learn about Words

1 _____ 6 _____

2 _____ 7 _____

3 _____ 8 _____

4 _____ 9 _____

5 _____ 10 _____

Number Correct [ ]

Think about It

D 1 _____ **E** 6 _____ **F** 11 _____

2 _____ 7 _____ 12 _____

3 _____ 8 _____ 13 _____

4 _____ 9 _____ 14 _____

5 _____ 10 _____ 15 _____

Number Correct [ ]

Record Page

Name _____ Date _____

Power Builder Color _____ Power Builder Number _____

A Comprehension

1 _____ 2 _____ 3 _____ 4 _____ 5 _____

Number Correct [＿＿]

B, C Learn about Words

1 _____   6 _____

2 _____   7 _____

3 _____   8 _____

4 _____   9 _____

5 _____   10 _____

Number Correct [＿＿]

Think about It

D 1 _____   **E** 6 _____   **F** 11 _____

2 _____   7 _____   12 _____

3 _____   8 _____   13 _____

4 _____   9 _____   14 _____

5 _____   10 _____   15 _____

Number Correct [＿＿]

Record Page

Name _____ Date _____

Power Builder Color _____ Power Builder Number _____

A Comprehension

1 _____ 2 _____ 3 _____ 4 _____ 5 _____

Number Correct ☐

B, C Learn about Words

1 _____ 6 _____

2 _____ 7 _____

3 _____ 8 _____

4 _____ 9 _____

5 _____ 10 _____

Number Correct ☐

Think about It

D1 _____ **E**6 _____ **F**11 _____

2 _____ 7 _____ 12 _____

3 _____ 8 _____ 13 _____

4 _____ 9 _____ 14 _____

5 _____ 10 _____ 15 _____

Number Correct ☐

Record Page

Name _____ Date _____

Power Builder Color _____ Power Builder Number _____

A Comprehension

1 _____ 2 _____ 3 _____ 4 _____ 5 _____

Number Correct [ ]

B, C Learn about Words

1 _____ 6 _____

2 _____ 7 _____

3 _____ 8 _____

4 _____ 9 _____

5 _____ 10 _____

Number Correct [ ]

Think about It

D1 _____ **E**6 _____ **F**11 _____

2 _____ 7 _____ 12 _____

3 _____ 8 _____ 13 _____

4 _____ 9 _____ 14 _____

5 _____ 10 _____ 15 _____

Number Correct [ ]

Record Page

Name _____ Date _____

Power Builder Color _____ Power Builder Number _____

A Comprehension

1 _____ 2 _____ 3 _____ 4 _____ 5 _____

Number Correct [   ]

B, C Learn about Words

1 _____   6 _____

2 _____   7 _____

3 _____   8 _____

4 _____   9 _____

5 _____   10 _____

Number Correct [   ]

Think about It

D 1 _____   **E** 6 _____   **F** 11 _____

2 _____   7 _____   12 _____

3 _____   8 _____   13 _____

4 _____   9 _____   14 _____

5 _____   10 _____   15 _____

Number Correct [   ]

Record Page

Name _____ Date _____

Power Builder Color _____ Power Builder Number _____

A Comprehension

1 _____ 2 _____ 3 _____ 4 _____ 5 _____

Number Correct [　　]

B, C Learn about Words

1 _____   6 _____

2 _____   7 _____

3 _____   8 _____

4 _____   9 _____

5 _____   10 _____

Number Correct [　　]

Think about It

D 1 _____   **E** 6 _____   **F** 11 _____

2 _____   7 _____   12 _____

3 _____   8 _____   13 _____

4 _____   9 _____   14 _____

5 _____   10 _____   15 _____

Number Correct [　　]

Record Page

Name _____ Date _____

Power Builder Color _____ Power Builder Number _____

A Comprehension

1 _____ 2 _____ 3 _____ 4 _____ 5 _____

Number Correct [ ]

B, C Learn about Words

1 _____ 6 _____

2 _____ 7 _____

3 _____ 8 _____

4 _____ 9 _____

5 _____ 10 _____

Number Correct [ ]

Think about It

D 1 _____ **E** 6 _____ **F** 11 _____

2 _____ 7 _____ 12 _____

3 _____ 8 _____ 13 _____

4 _____ 9 _____ 14 _____

5 _____ 10 _____ 15 _____

Number Correct [ ]

Record Page

Name _____ Date _____

Power Builder Color _____ Power Builder Number _____

A Comprehension

1 _____ 2 _____ 3 _____ 4 _____ 5 _____

Number Correct [ ]

B, C Learn about Words

1 _____ 6 _____

2 _____ 7 _____

3 _____ 8 _____

4 _____ 9 _____

5 _____ 10 _____

Number Correct [ ]

Think about It

D 1 _____ **E** 6 _____ **F** 11 _____

2 _____ 7 _____ 12 _____

3 _____ 8 _____ 13 _____

4 _____ 9 _____ 14 _____

5 _____ 10 _____ 15 _____

Number Correct [ ]

Record Page

Name _____ Date _____

Power Builder Color _____ Power Builder Number _____

A Comprehension

1 _____ 2 _____ 3 _____ 4 _____ 5 _____

Number Correct ☐

B, C Learn about Words

1 _____ 6 _____

2 _____ 7 _____

3 _____ 8 _____

4 _____ 9 _____

5 _____ 10 _____

Number Correct ☐

Think about It

D 1 _____ **E** 6 _____ **F** 11 _____

2 _____ 7 _____ 12 _____

3 _____ 8 _____ 13 _____

4 _____ 9 _____ 14 _____

5 _____ 10 _____ 15 _____

Number Correct ☐

Record Page

Name _____ Date _____

Power Builder Color _____ Power Builder Number _____

A Comprehension

1 _____ 2 _____ 3 _____ 4 _____ 5 _____

Number Correct [ ]

B, C Learn about Words

1 _____ 6 _____

2 _____ 7 _____

3 _____ 8 _____

4 _____ 9 _____

5 _____ 10 _____

Number Correct [ ]

Think about It

D 1 _____ **E** 6 _____ **F** 11 _____

2 _____ 7 _____ 12 _____

3 _____ 8 _____ 13 _____

4 _____ 9 _____ 14 _____

5 _____ 10 _____ 15 _____

Number Correct [ ]

Record Page

Name _____ Date _____

Power Builder Color _____ Power Builder Number _____

A Comprehension

1 _____ 2 _____ 3 _____ 4 _____ 5 _____

Number Correct [___]

B, C Learn about Words

1 _____ 6 _____

2 _____ 7 _____

3 _____ 8 _____

4 _____ 9 _____

5 _____ 10 _____

Number Correct [___]

Think about It

D 1 _____ **E** 6 _____ **F** 11 _____

2 _____ 7 _____ 12 _____

3 _____ 8 _____ 13 _____

4 _____ 9 _____ 14 _____

5 _____ 10 _____ 15 _____

Number Correct [___]

Record Page

Name _____   Date _____

Power Builder Color _____   Power Builder Number _____

A Comprehension

1 _____ 2 _____ 3 _____ 4 _____ 5 _____

Number Correct [   ]

B, C Learn about Words

1 _____   6 _____

2 _____   7 _____

3 _____   8 _____

4 _____   9 _____

5 _____   10 _____

Number Correct [   ]

Think about It

D 1 _____   **E** 6 _____   **F** 11 _____

2 _____   7 _____   12 _____

3 _____   8 _____   13 _____

4 _____   9 _____   14 _____

5 _____   10 _____   15 _____

Number Correct [   ]

Record Page

Name _____   Date _____

Power Builder Color _____   Power Builder Number _____

A Comprehension

1 _____ 2 _____ 3 _____ 4 _____ 5 _____

Number Correct [ ]

B, C Learn about Words

1 _____   6 _____

2 _____   7 _____

3 _____   8 _____

4 _____   9 _____

5 _____   10 _____

Number Correct [ ]

Think about It

D 1 _____   **E** 6 _____   **F** 11 _____

2 _____   7 _____   12 _____

3 _____   8 _____   13 _____

4 _____   9 _____   14 _____

5 _____   10 _____   15 _____

Number Correct [ ]

Record Page

Name _____ Date _____

Power Builder Color _____ Power Builder Number _____

A Comprehension

1 _____ 2 _____ 3 _____ 4 _____ 5 _____

Number Correct ☐

B, C Learn about Words

1 _____ 6 _____

2 _____ 7 _____

3 _____ 8 _____

4 _____ 9 _____

5 _____ 10 _____

Number Correct ☐

Think about It

D 1 _____ **E** 6 _____ **F** 11 _____

2 _____ 7 _____ 12 _____

3 _____ 8 _____ 13 _____

4 _____ 9 _____ 14 _____

5 _____ 10 _____ 15 _____

Number Correct ☐

Record Page

Name _____ Date _____

Power Builder Color _____ Power Builder Number _____

A Comprehension

1 _____ 2 _____ 3 _____ 4 _____ 5 _____

Number Correct [   ]

B, C Learn about Words

1 _____   6 _____

2 _____   7 _____

3 _____   8 _____

4 _____   9 _____

5 _____   10 _____

Number Correct [   ]

Think about It

D1 _____   **E**6 _____   **F**11 _____

2 _____   7 _____   12 _____

3 _____   8 _____   13 _____

4 _____   9 _____   14 _____

5 _____   10 _____   15 _____

Number Correct [   ]

Record Page

Name _____ Date _____

Power Builder Color _____ Power Builder Number _____

A Comprehension

1 _____ 2 _____ 3 _____ 4 _____ 5 _____

Number Correct [   ]

B, C Learn about Words

1 _____ 6 _____

2 _____ 7 _____

3 _____ 8 _____

4 _____ 9 _____

5 _____ 10 _____

Number Correct [   ]

Think about It

D 1 _____ **E** 6 _____ **F** 11 _____

2 _____ 7 _____ 12 _____

3 _____ 8 _____ 13 _____

4 _____ 9 _____ 14 _____

5 _____ 10 _____ 15 _____

Number Correct [   ]

Record Page

Name _____   Date _____

Power Builder Color _____   Power Builder Number _____

A Comprehension

1 _____ 2 _____ 3 _____ 4 _____ 5 _____

Number Correct [ ]

B, C Learn about Words

1 _____   6 _____

2 _____   7 _____

3 _____   8 _____

4 _____   9 _____

5 _____   10 _____

Number Correct [ ]

Think about It

D 1 _____   **E** 6 _____   **F** 11 _____

2 _____   7 _____   12 _____

3 _____   8 _____   13 _____

4 _____   9 _____   14 _____

5 _____   10 _____   15 _____

Number Correct [ ]

Record Page

Name _____ Date _____

Power Builder Color _____ Power Builder Number _____

A Comprehension

1 _____ 2 _____ 3 _____ 4 _____ 5 _____

Number Correct [   ]

B, C Learn about Words

1 _____ 6 _____

2 _____ 7 _____

3 _____ 8 _____

4 _____ 9 _____

5 _____ 10 _____

Number Correct [   ]

Think about It

D 1 _____ **E** 6 _____ **F** 11 _____

2 _____ 7 _____ 12 _____

3 _____ 8 _____ 13 _____

4 _____ 9 _____ 14 _____

5 _____ 10 _____ 15 _____

Number Correct [   ]

Power Builder Number	Date

My Reading Progress Chart: ORANGE LEVEL

Fill in a box for every correct answer on your Power Builder.

A Comprehension

1	2	3	4	5
1	2	3	4	5
1	2	3	4	5
1	2	3	4	5
1	2	3	4	5
1	2	3	4	5
1	2	3	4	5
1	2	3	4	5
1	2	3	4	5
1	2	3	4	5
1	2	3	4	5
1	2	3	4	5
1	2	3	4	5

B, C Learn about Words

1	2	3	4	5	6	7	8	9	10
1	2	3	4	5	6	7	8	9	10
1	2	3	4	5	6	7	8	9	10
1	2	3	4	5	6	7	8	9	10
1	2	3	4	5	6	7	8	9	10
1	2	3	4	5	6	7	8	9	10
1	2	3	4	5	6	7	8	9	10
1	2	3	4	5	6	7	8	9	10
1	2	3	4	5	6	7	8	9	10
1	2	3	4	5	6	7	8	9	10
1	2	3	4	5	6	7	8	9	10
1	2	3	4	5	6	7	8	9	10

D Think about It

1	2	3	4	5
1	2	3	4	5
1	2	3	4	5
1	2	3	4	5
1	2	3	4	5
1	2	3	4	5
1	2	3	4	5
1	2	3	4	5
1	2	3	4	5
1	2	3	4	5
1	2	3	4	5
1	2	3	4	5

My Reading Progress Chart: GOLD LEVEL

Fill in a box for every correct answer on your Power Builder.

A Comprehension **B, C** Learn about Words **D** Think about It

Power Builder Number	Date	A Comprehension	B, C Learn about Words	D Think about It
		1 2 3 4 5	1 2 3 4 5 6 7 8 9 10	1 2 3 4 5
		1 2 3 4 5	1 2 3 4 5 6 7 8 9 10	1 2 3 4 5
		1 2 3 4 5	1 2 3 4 5 6 7 8 9 10	1 2 3 4 5
		1 2 3 4 5	1 2 3 4 5 6 7 8 9 10	1 2 3 4 5
		1 2 3 4 5	1 2 3 4 5 6 7 8 9 10	1 2 3 4 5
		1 2 3 4 5	1 2 3 4 5 6 7 8 9 10	1 2 3 4 5
		1 2 3 4 5	1 2 3 4 5 6 7 8 9 10	1 2 3 4 5
		1 2 3 4 5	1 2 3 4 5 6 7 8 9 10	1 2 3 4 5
		1 2 3 4 5	1 2 3 4 5 6 7 8 9 10	1 2 3 4 5
		1 2 3 4 5	1 2 3 4 5 6 7 8 9 10	1 2 3 4 5
		1 2 3 4 5	1 2 3 4 5 6 7 8 9 10	1 2 3 4 5
		1 2 3 4 5	1 2 3 4 5 6 7 8 9 10	1 2 3 4 5

117

My Reading Progress Chart: BROWN LEVEL

Fill in a box for every correct answer on your Power Builder.

Power Builder Number	Date	A Comprehension	B, C Learn about Words	D Think about It
		1 2 3 4 5	1 2 3 4 5 6 7 8 9 10	1 2 3 4 5
		1 2 3 4 5	1 2 3 4 5 6 7 8 9 10	1 2 3 4 5
		1 2 3 4 5	1 2 3 4 5 6 7 8 9 10	1 2 3 4 5
		1 2 3 4 5	1 2 3 4 5 6 7 8 9 10	1 2 3 4 5
		1 2 3 4 5	1 2 3 4 5 6 7 8 9 10	1 2 3 4 5
		1 2 3 4 5	1 2 3 4 5 6 7 8 9 10	1 2 3 4 5
		1 2 3 4 5	1 2 3 4 5 6 7 8 9 10	1 2 3 4 5
		1 2 3 4 5	1 2 3 4 5 6 7 8 9 10	1 2 3 4 5
		1 2 3 4 5	1 2 3 4 5 6 7 8 9 10	1 2 3 4 5
		1 2 3 4 5	1 2 3 4 5 6 7 8 9 10	1 2 3 4 5
		1 2 3 4 5	1 2 3 4 5 6 7 8 9 10	1 2 3 4 5
		1 2 3 4 5	1 2 3 4 5 6 7 8 9 10	1 2 3 4 5

My Reading Progress Chart: TAN LEVEL

Fill in a box for every correct answer on your Power Builder.

Power Builder Number	Date	A Comprehension	B, C Learn about Words	D, E Think about It
		1 2 3 4 5	1 2 3 4 5 6 7 8 9 10	1 2 3 4 5 6 7 8 9 10
		1 2 3 4 5	1 2 3 4 5 6 7 8 9 10	1 2 3 4 5 6 7 8 9 10
		1 2 3 4 5	1 2 3 4 5 6 7 8 9 10	1 2 3 4 5 6 7 8 9 10
		1 2 3 4 5	1 2 3 4 5 6 7 8 9 10	1 2 3 4 5 6 7 8 9 10
		1 2 3 4 5	1 2 3 4 5 6 7 8 9 10	1 2 3 4 5 6 7 8 9 10
		1 2 3 4 5	1 2 3 4 5 6 7 8 9 10	1 2 3 4 5 6 7 8 9 10
		1 2 3 4 5	1 2 3 4 5 6 7 8 9 10	1 2 3 4 5 6 7 8 9 10
		1 2 3 4 5	1 2 3 4 5 6 7 8 9 10	1 2 3 4 5 6 7 8 9 10
		1 2 3 4 5	1 2 3 4 5 6 7 8 9 10	1 2 3 4 5 6 7 8 9 10
		1 2 3 4 5	1 2 3 4 5 6 7 8 9 10	1 2 3 4 5 6 7 8 9 10
		1 2 3 4 5	1 2 3 4 5 6 7 8 9 10	1 2 3 4 5 6 7 8 9 10
		1 2 3 4 5	1 2 3 4 5 6 7 8 9 10	1 2 3 4 5 6 7 8 9 10

My Reading Progress Chart: LIME LEVEL

Fill in a box for every correct answer on your Power Builder.

Power Builder Number	Date	A Comprehension	B, C Learn about Words	D, E Think about It
		1 2 3 4 5	1 2 3 4 5 6 7 8 9 10	1 2 3 4 5 6 7 8 9 10
		1 2 3 4 5	1 2 3 4 5 6 7 8 9 10	1 2 3 4 5 6 7 8 9 10
		1 2 3 4 5	1 2 3 4 5 6 7 8 9 10	1 2 3 4 5 6 7 8 9 10
		1 2 3 4 5	1 2 3 4 5 6 7 8 9 10	1 2 3 4 5 6 7 8 9 10
		1 2 3 4 5	1 2 3 4 5 6 7 8 9 10	1 2 3 4 5 6 7 8 9 10
		1 2 3 4 5	1 2 3 4 5 6 7 8 9 10	1 2 3 4 5 6 7 8 9 10
		1 2 3 4 5	1 2 3 4 5 6 7 8 9 10	1 2 3 4 5 6 7 8 9 10
		1 2 3 4 5	1 2 3 4 5 6 7 8 9 10	1 2 3 4 5 6 7 8 9 10
		1 2 3 4 5	1 2 3 4 5 6 7 8 9 10	1 2 3 4 5 6 7 8 9 10
		1 2 3 4 5	1 2 3 4 5 6 7 8 9 10	1 2 3 4 5 6 7 8 9 10
		1 2 3 4 5	1 2 3 4 5 6 7 8 9 10	1 2 3 4 5 6 7 8 9 10
		1 2 3 4 5	1 2 3 4 5 6 7 8 9 10	1 2 3 4 5 6 7 8 9 10

My Reading Progress Chart: GREEN LEVEL

Fill in a box for every correct answer on your Power Builder.

Power Builder Number	Date	A Comprehension					B, C Learn about Words										D, E Think about It									
		1	2	3	4	5	1	2	3	4	5	6	7	8	9	10	1	2	3	4	5	6	7	8	9	10
		1	2	3	4	5	1	2	3	4	5	6	7	8	9	10	1	2	3	4	5	6	7	8	9	10
		1	2	3	4	5	1	2	3	4	5	6	7	8	9	10	1	2	3	4	5	6	7	8	9	10
		1	2	3	4	5	1	2	3	4	5	6	7	8	9	10	1	2	3	4	5	6	7	8	9	10
		1	2	3	4	5	1	2	3	4	5	6	7	8	9	10	1	2	3	4	5	6	7	8	9	10
		1	2	3	4	5	1	2	3	4	5	6	7	8	9	10	1	2	3	4	5	6	7	8	9	10
		1	2	3	4	5	1	2	3	4	5	6	7	8	9	10	1	2	3	4	5	6	7	8	9	10
		1	2	3	4	5	1	2	3	4	5	6	7	8	9	10	1	2	3	4	5	6	7	8	9	10
		1	2	3	4	5	1	2	3	4	5	6	7	8	9	10	1	2	3	4	5	6	7	8	9	10
		1	2	3	4	5	1	2	3	4	5	6	7	8	9	10	1	2	3	4	5	6	7	8	9	10
		1	2	3	4	5	1	2	3	4	5	6	7	8	9	10	1	2	3	4	5	6	7	8	9	10
		1	2	3	4	5	1	2	3	4	5	6	7	8	9	10	1	2	3	4	5	6	7	8	9	10

My Reading Progress Chart: AQUA LEVEL

Fill in a box for every correct answer on your Power Builder.

Power Builder Number	Date

A Comprehension

1	2	3	4	5
1	2	3	4	5
1	2	3	4	5
1	2	3	4	5
1	2	3	4	5
1	2	3	4	5
1	2	3	4	5
1	2	3	4	5
1	2	3	4	5
1	2	3	4	5
1	2	3	4	5

B, C Learn about Words

1	2	3	4	5	6	7	8	9	10
1	2	3	4	5	6	7	8	9	10
1	2	3	4	5	6	7	8	9	10
1	2	3	4	5	6	7	8	9	10
1	2	3	4	5	6	7	8	9	10
1	2	3	4	5	6	7	8	9	10
1	2	3	4	5	6	7	8	9	10
1	2	3	4	5	6	7	8	9	10
1	2	3	4	5	6	7	8	9	10
1	2	3	4	5	6	7	8	9	10
1	2	3	4	5	6	7	8	9	10

D, E Think about It

1	2	3	4	5	6	7	8	9	10
1	2	3	4	5	6	7	8	9	10
1	2	3	4	5	6	7	8	9	10
1	2	3	4	5	6	7	8	9	10
1	2	3	4	5	6	7	8	9	10
1	2	3	4	5	6	7	8	9	10
1	2	3	4	5	6	7	8	9	10
1	2	3	4	5	6	7	8	9	10
1	2	3	4	5	6	7	8	9	10
1	2	3	4	5	6	7	8	9	10
1	2	3	4	5	6	7	8	9	10

My Reading Progress Chart: BLUE LEVEL

Fill in a box for every correct answer on your Power Builder.

Power Builder Number	Date	A Comprehension	B, C Learn about Words	D, E Think about It
		1 2 3 4 5	1 2 3 4 5 6 7 8 9 10	1 2 3 4 5 6 7 8 9 10
		1 2 3 4 5	1 2 3 4 5 6 7 8 9 10	1 2 3 4 5 6 7 8 9 10
		1 2 3 4 5	1 2 3 4 5 6 7 8 9 10	1 2 3 4 5 6 7 8 9 10
		1 2 3 4 5	1 2 3 4 5 6 7 8 9 10	1 2 3 4 5 6 7 8 9 10
		1 2 3 4 5	1 2 3 4 5 6 7 8 9 10	1 2 3 4 5 6 7 8 9 10
		1 2 3 4 5	1 2 3 4 5 6 7 8 9 10	1 2 3 4 5 6 7 8 9 10
		1 2 3 4 5	1 2 3 4 5 6 7 8 9 10	1 2 3 4 5 6 7 8 9 10
		1 2 3 4 5	1 2 3 4 5 6 7 8 9 10	1 2 3 4 5 6 7 8 9 10
		1 2 3 4 5	1 2 3 4 5 6 7 8 9 10	1 2 3 4 5 6 7 8 9 10
		1 2 3 4 5	1 2 3 4 5 6 7 8 9 10	1 2 3 4 5 6 7 8 9 10
		1 2 3 4 5	1 2 3 4 5 6 7 8 9 10	1 2 3 4 5 6 7 8 9 10
		1 2 3 4 5	1 2 3 4 5 6 7 8 9 10	1 2 3 4 5 6 7 8 9 10

My Reading Progress Chart: PURPLE LEVEL

Fill in a box for every correct answer on your Power Builder.

Power Builder Number		Date

A Comprehension

Each row: 1 2 3 4 5

B, C Learn about Words

Each row: 1 2 3 4 5 6 7 8 9 10

D, E, F Think about It

Each row: 1 2 3 4 5 6 7 8 9 10 11 12 13 14 15

My Reading Progress Chart: VIOLET LEVEL

Fill in a box for every correct answer on your Power Builder.

Power Builder Number	Date	A Comprehension	B, C Learn about Words	D, E, F Think about It
		1 2 3 4 5	1 2 3 4 5 6 7 8 9 10	1 2 3 4 5 6 7 8 9 10 11 12 13 14 15
		1 2 3 4 5	1 2 3 4 5 6 7 8 9 10	1 2 3 4 5 6 7 8 9 10 11 12 13 14 15
		1 2 3 4 5	1 2 3 4 5 6 7 8 9 10	1 2 3 4 5 6 7 8 9 10 11 12 13 14 15
		1 2 3 4 5	1 2 3 4 5 6 7 8 9 10	1 2 3 4 5 6 7 8 9 10 11 12 13 14 15
		1 2 3 4 5	1 2 3 4 5 6 7 8 9 10	1 2 3 4 5 6 7 8 9 10 11 12 13 14 15
		1 2 3 4 5	1 2 3 4 5 6 7 8 9 10	1 2 3 4 5 6 7 8 9 10 11 12 13 14 15
		1 2 3 4 5	1 2 3 4 5 6 7 8 9 10	1 2 3 4 5 6 7 8 9 10 11 12 13 14 15
		1 2 3 4 5	1 2 3 4 5 6 7 8 9 10	1 2 3 4 5 6 7 8 9 10 11 12 13 14 15
		1 2 3 4 5	1 2 3 4 5 6 7 8 9 10	1 2 3 4 5 6 7 8 9 10 11 12 13 14 15
		1 2 3 4 5	1 2 3 4 5 6 7 8 9 10	1 2 3 4 5 6 7 8 9 10 11 12 13 14 15
		1 2 3 4 5	1 2 3 4 5 6 7 8 9 10	1 2 3 4 5 6 7 8 9 10 11 12 13 14 15
		1 2 3 4 5	1 2 3 4 5 6 7 8 9 10	1 2 3 4 5 6 7 8 9 10 11 12 13 14 15

My Reading Progress Chart: ROSE LEVEL

Fill in a box for every correct answer on your Power Builder.

Power Builder Number	Date	A Comprehension					B, C Learn about Words										D, E, F Think about It														
		1	2	3	4	5	1	2	3	4	5	6	7	8	9	10	1	2	3	4	5	6	7	8	9	10	11	12	13	14	15
		1	2	3	4	5	1	2	3	4	5	6	7	8	9	10	1	2	3	4	5	6	7	8	9	10	11	12	13	14	15
		1	2	3	4	5	1	2	3	4	5	6	7	8	9	10	1	2	3	4	5	6	7	8	9	10	11	12	13	14	15
		1	2	3	4	5	1	2	3	4	5	6	7	8	9	10	1	2	3	4	5	6	7	8	9	10	11	12	13	14	15
		1	2	3	4	5	1	2	3	4	5	6	7	8	9	10	1	2	3	4	5	6	7	8	9	10	11	12	13	14	15
		1	2	3	4	5	1	2	3	4	5	6	7	8	9	10	1	2	3	4	5	6	7	8	9	10	11	12	13	14	15
		1	2	3	4	5	1	2	3	4	5	6	7	8	9	10	1	2	3	4	5	6	7	8	9	10	11	12	13	14	15
		1	2	3	4	5	1	2	3	4	5	6	7	8	9	10	1	2	3	4	5	6	7	8	9	10	11	12	13	14	15
		1	2	3	4	5	1	2	3	4	5	6	7	8	9	10	1	2	3	4	5	6	7	8	9	10	11	12	13	14	15
		1	2	3	4	5	1	2	3	4	5	6	7	8	9	10	1	2	3	4	5	6	7	8	9	10	11	12	13	14	15
		1	2	3	4	5	1	2	3	4	5	6	7	8	9	10	1	2	3	4	5	6	7	8	9	10	11	12	13	14	15
		1	2	3	4	5	1	2	3	4	5	6	7	8	9	10	1	2	3	4	5	6	7	8	9	10	11	12	13	14	15

My Reading Progress Chart: RED LEVEL

Fill in a box for every correct answer on your Power Builder.

Power Builder Number	Date	A Comprehension	B, C Learn about Words	D, E, F Think about It
		1 2 3 4 5	1 2 3 4 5 6 7 8 9 10	1 2 3 4 5 6 7 8 9 10 11 12 13 14 15
		1 2 3 4 5	1 2 3 4 5 6 7 8 9 10	1 2 3 4 5 6 7 8 9 10 11 12 13 14 15
		1 2 3 4 5	1 2 3 4 5 6 7 8 9 10	1 2 3 4 5 6 7 8 9 10 11 12 13 14 15
		1 2 3 4 5	1 2 3 4 5 6 7 8 9 10	1 2 3 4 5 6 7 8 9 10 11 12 13 14 15
		1 2 3 4 5	1 2 3 4 5 6 7 8 9 10	1 2 3 4 5 6 7 8 9 10 11 12 13 14 15
		1 2 3 4 5	1 2 3 4 5 6 7 8 9 10	1 2 3 4 5 6 7 8 9 10 11 12 13 14 15
		1 2 3 4 5	1 2 3 4 5 6 7 8 9 10	1 2 3 4 5 6 7 8 9 10 11 12 13 14 15
		1 2 3 4 5	1 2 3 4 5 6 7 8 9 10	1 2 3 4 5 6 7 8 9 10 11 12 13 14 15
		1 2 3 4 5	1 2 3 4 5 6 7 8 9 10	1 2 3 4 5 6 7 8 9 10 11 12 13 14 15
		1 2 3 4 5	1 2 3 4 5 6 7 8 9 10	1 2 3 4 5 6 7 8 9 10 11 12 13 14 15
		1 2 3 4 5	1 2 3 4 5 6 7 8 9 10	1 2 3 4 5 6 7 8 9 10 11 12 13 14 15
		1 2 3 4 5	1 2 3 4 5 6 7 8 9 10	1 2 3 4 5 6 7 8 9 10 11 12 13 14 15
		1 2 3 4 5	1 2 3 4 5 6 7 8 9 10	1 2 3 4 5 6 7 8 9 10 11 12 13 14 15

Answer Keys

Starter 1–Orange

Comprehension
A
1 a
2 a
3 b
4 b
5 a

Learn about Words
B
1 grow
2 know
3 snow
4 row
5 crow

C
6 know
7 grow
8 crow
9 snow
10 row

Think about It
D
1 b
2 a
3 b
4 a
5 a

Starter 2–Orange

Comprehension
A
1 a
2 a
3 b
4 b
5 b

Learn about Words
B
1 mat
2 that
3 fat
4 sat
5 cat

C
6 sat
7 cat
8 that
9 fat
10 mat

Think about It
D
1 No
2 Yes
3 No
4 Yes
5 No

Starter 3–Gold

Comprehension
A
1 b
2 b
3 a
4 a
5 a

Learn about Words
B
1 day
2 stay
3 play
4 way
5 may

C
6 play
7 way
8 may
9 stay
10 day

Think about It
D
1 b
2 b
3 a
4 b
5 a

Starter 4–Tan

Comprehension
A
1 b
2 a
3 a
4 b
5 b

Learn about Words
B
1 students
2 words
3 worms
4 spoonerisms
5 mothers

C
6 words
7 worms
8 students
9 mothers
10 spoonerisms

Think about It
D
1 b
2 a
3 a
4 a
5 b

E
6 walked
7 sold
8 what
9 friend
10 said

Starter 5–Green

Comprehension
A
1 b
2 a
3 b
4 a
5 a

Learn about Words
B
1 invite
2 room
3 find
4 met
5 park

C
6 invite
7 find
8 room
9 park
10 met

Think about It
D
1 hot
2 turtle
3 mouse
4 cool
5 white

E
6 girlfriend
7 swimsuit
8 sunglasses
9 houseboat
10 catfish

Starter 6–Blue

Comprehension
A
1 c
2 a
3 b
4 a
5 a

Learn about Words
B
1 blanket
2 cupboard
3 shrank
4 scissors
5 sewed
6 scarf
7 package
8 special

C
9 b
10 a

Think about It
D
1 middle
2 middle
3 beginning
4 end
5 beginning

E
6 did not
7 could not
8 Do not
9 Here is
10 I will

STRATEGY LESSON 2

1 a
2 b
3 b
4 b